INTERMITTENT FASTING FOR WOMEN OVER 50

Your Guide to Safe and Sustainable Weight Loss and Menopause Symptom Relief

By

Hector Wiggins

Table of Contents

CHAPTER ONE

INTRODUCTION

Welcome to "Intermittent Fasting for Women over 50," where we start on a transformative progress towards reclaiming health, vitality, and empowerment in the golden years of life. As women enter their 50s and beyond, they are often confronted with a myriad of unique challenges that can impact their overall health and wellbeing. From overcoming the hormonal fluctuations of menopause to grappling with the effects of aging on metabolism and energy levels, the road to optimal health can feel like an uphill battle.

In this pivotal stage of life, many women find themselves facing unwelcome changes such as weight gain, decreased energy, and hormonal imbalances, which can significantly impact their quality of life. Traditional approaches to diet and exercise may no longer yield the same results, leaving many feeling frustrated and discouraged.

However, amidst these challenges lies a powerful solution that has the potential to revolutionize the way women over 50 approach their health: intermittent fasting. Far more than just a passing fad, intermittent fasting has emerged as a scientifically-backed strategy that offers a multitude of benefits uniquely suited to the needs of women in this age group.

By strategically timing periods of eating and fasting, intermittent fasting offers a holistic approach to health that addresses the root causes of many age-related issues. From promoting weight loss and improving metabolic health to enhancing mental clarity and reducing the risk of chronic diseases, the benefits of intermittent fasting are vast and far-reaching.

But perhaps most importantly, intermittent fasting empowers women to take control of their health and reclaim their vitality in a way that is sustainable and empowering. By embracing this lifestyle approach, women over 50 have the opportunity to not only improve their physical health but also cultivate a sense of confidence and empowerment that transcends age.

In this comprehensive guide, we will explore the science behind intermittent fasting, analyze various fasting protocols customized specifically to the needs of women over 50, and provide practical tips for incorporating intermittent fasting into daily life. Whether you're looking to shed unwanted pounds, boost your energy levels, or simply feel your best as you age, this guide will serve as your roadmap to success.

So join us as we start on this transformative
progress together, and discover how intermittent
fasting can be the game-changer you've been
searching for in your quest for optimal health and
wellbeing. It's time to take control of your health,
embrace your inner strength, and thrive in this new
chapter of life.

What is Intermittent Fasting?

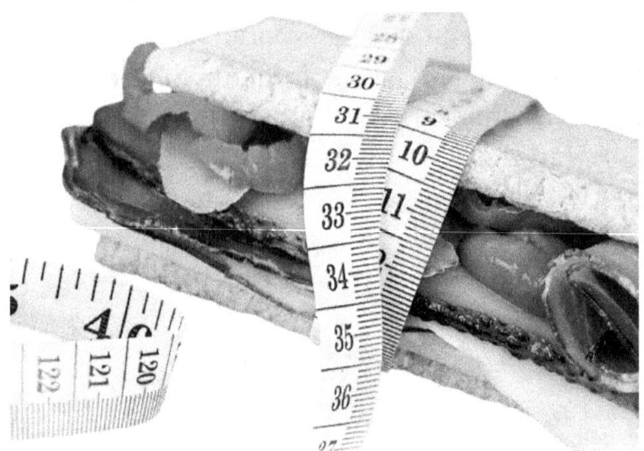

A dietary pattern known as intermittent fasting (IF) alternates between times when one eats and when one fasts. Unlike traditional diets that focus on what you eat, intermittent fasting places emphasis on when you eat. This approach has gained significant popularity in recent years, not only for its potential weight loss benefits but also for its purported effects on overall health and longevity.

At its core, intermittent fasting is a simple concept with profound implications for human health. Rather than restricting specific foods or counting calories, intermittent fasting involves cycling between periods of eating and fasting. There are several different methods of intermittent fasting, but they all share the common goal of extending the period of time between meals.

One of the most popular methods of intermittent fasting is the 16/8 method, which involves fasting for 16 hours each day and restricting eating to an 8-hour window. Another common approach is the 5:2 method, which involves eating normally for five days of the week and significantly reducing calorie intake (typically to around 500-600 calories) on the remaining two days. There are also variations such as alternate-day fasting, where individuals alternate between days of normal eating and fasting, and the eat-stop-eat method, which involves fasting for a full 24 hours once or twice a week.

The ease of use and adaptability of intermittent fasting are its main draws. Unlike many traditional diets that require strict adherence to specific meal plans or food restrictions, intermittent fasting can be adapted to fit individual lifestyles and preferences. Additionally, intermittent fasting has been shown to offer a variety of potential health benefits beyond weight loss. Research suggests that intermittent fasting may help improve metabolic health, regulate blood sugar levels, reduce inflammation, and even enhance brain function.

One of the key mechanisms behind the benefits of intermittent fasting is thought to be its effect on cellular repair processes and hormone regulation. During fasting periods, the body undergoes a series of metabolic changes that promote fat burning and cellular repair. Additionally, fasting has been shown to stimulate the production of certain hormones, such as human growth hormone (HGH), which plays a role in muscle growth, fat loss, and overall health.

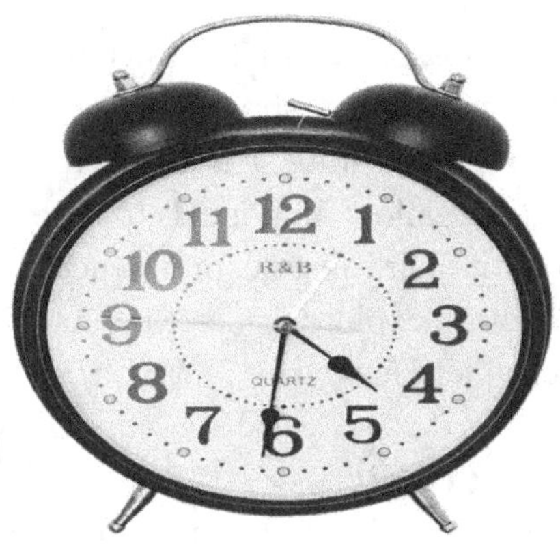

Overall, intermittent fasting represents a shift away from traditional dieting paradigms towards a more holistic approach to health and wellness. By harnessing the body's natural ability to adapt to periods of food scarcity, intermittent fasting offers a unique and potentially powerful tool for improving health, optimizing metabolism, and promoting longevity.

Types of Intermittent Fasting

Intermittent fasting encompasses a variety of fasting methods, each with its own unique approach to cycling between periods of eating and fasting. These different types of intermittent fasting allow individuals to tailor their fasting regimen to fit their lifestyle, preferences, and health goals. Here, we'll explore some of the most common types of intermittent fasting:

Time-Restricted Eating (TRE):
Time-restricted eating involves limiting your daily eating window to a specific period of time, typically ranging from 4 to 10 hours, followed by a fasting period for the remainder of the day. The 16/8 method, for example, restricts eating to an 8-hour window (e.g., 12:00 pm to 8:00 pm) with fasting during the remaining 16 hours.

Alternate-Day Fasting (ADF):
Alternate-day fasting involves alternating between days of normal eating and fasting. On fasting days, calorie intake is significantly reduced or eliminated altogether, while on non-fasting days, individuals can eat freely. Modified alternate-day fasting allows for some calorie consumption (usually around 500 calories) on fasting days to make the regimen more sustainable.

5:2 Method:
The 5:2 method involves eating normally for five days of the week and restricting calorie intake to around 500-600 calories on two non-consecutive fasting days. This approach allows for flexibility in food choices and meal timing on non-fasting days.

Eat-Stop-Eat:
Eat-stop-eat refers to a once or twice-weekly complete 24-hour fast. For example, individuals may choose to fast from dinner one day until dinner the following day. This method is straightforward but may be challenging for some people to adhere to due to the longer fasting periods.

Extended Fasting:
Extended fasting involves fasting for periods longer than 24 hours, often ranging from 48 to 72 hours or even longer. Extended fasts may be conducted occasionally for detoxification purposes or as part of a religious or spiritual practice. However, they require careful planning and supervision to ensure adequate hydration and nutrient intake.

Each type of intermittent fasting has its own benefits and challenges, and the best approach may vary from person to person. It's essential to consider factors such as individual health status, lifestyle, and goals when choosing an intermittent fasting regimen. Experimenting with different methods and finding what works best for you can help maximize the benefits of intermittent fasting while ensuring it remains sustainable and enjoyable in the long term.

Benefits of Intermittent Fasting for Women Over 50

Intermittent fasting offers a multitude of potential benefits for women over 50, addressing many of the unique health challenges they may face during this stage of life. Here's a comprehensive look at the benefits of intermittent fasting for women over 50:

Weight Management:
Intermittent fasting can be an effective tool for weight management in women over 50. By reducing calorie intake and promoting fat burning, intermittent fasting may help women achieve and maintain a healthy weight, which is paramount for overall health and wellbeing.

Improved Metabolic Health:
Aging can lead to changes in metabolism, including decreased insulin sensitivity and increased risk of metabolic disorders such as type 2 diabetes. Intermittent fasting has been shown to improve insulin sensitivity, regulate blood sugar levels, and reduce the risk of insulin resistance and diabetes in women over 50.

Enhanced Brain Function:
There is evidence that intermittent fasting enhances brain health and cognitive performance. By promoting the production of brain-derived neurotrophic factor (BDNF) and enhancing synaptic plasticity, intermittent fasting may help protect against age-related cognitive decline and improve memory and learning abilities in women over 50.

Increased Energy Levels:
Many women over 50 experience decreased energy levels and fatigue, which can impact their quality of life. Intermittent fasting has been shown to increase energy levels by enhancing mitochondrial function and improving cellular energy production, helping women feel more energetic and alert throughout the day.

Hormonal Balance:
Hormonal changes associated with menopause can lead to symptoms such as hot flashes, mood swings, and sleep disturbances. Intermittent fasting has been found to regulate hormone levels, including insulin, leptin, and ghrelin, which may help alleviate menopausal symptoms and promote hormonal balance in women over 50.

Reduced Inflammation:
Chronic inflammation is a common feature of aging and is associated with a variety of age-related diseases, including cardiovascular disease, arthritis, and Alzheimer's disease. Intermittent fasting has been shown to reduce inflammation markers in the body, potentially lowering the risk of age-related inflammatory conditions in women over 50.

Heart Health:
Intermittent fasting may have beneficial effects on heart health by reducing risk factors such as high blood pressure, cholesterol levels, and triglycerides. By promoting weight loss, improving insulin sensitivity, and reducing inflammation, intermittent fasting may help lower the risk of cardiovascular disease in women over 50.

Longevity:
Emerging research suggests that intermittent fasting may extend lifespan and promote longevity by activating cellular repair processes, enhancing stress resistance, and increasing the production of anti-aging proteins. By promoting overall health and resilience, intermittent fasting may help women over 50 live longer, healthier lives.

Intermittent Fasting (IF) Principles for Women Over 50

Intermittent fasting (IF) principles for women over 50 involve tailoring fasting protocols to address the unique needs and challenges associated with this stage of life. Here are the key principles to consider when implementing intermittent fasting for women over 50:

Consultation with Healthcare Provider:
Before starting any fasting regimen, it's essential for women over 50 to consult with their healthcare provider, especially if they have underlying health conditions or are taking medications. A healthcare provider can help assess individual health status and provide guidance on the safety and suitability of intermittent fasting.

Customized Approach:
Recognizing that women over 50 may have different nutritional needs and health concerns compared to younger individuals, intermittent fasting should be approached with customization in mind. Tailoring fasting protocols to accommodate factors such as hormonal changes, metabolic rate, and activity levels can optimize the benefits of intermittent fasting for women in this age group.

Gradual Implementation:
Intermittent fasting should be introduced gradually to allow the body to adapt to the fasting and feeding cycles. Starting with shorter fasting periods and gradually increasing fasting duration over time can help minimize potential side effects and promote long-term adherence to the fasting regimen.

Focus on Nutrient-Dense Foods:
During eating windows, women over 50 should prioritize nutrient-dense foods to ensure adequate intake of essential nutrients, vitamins, and minerals. Emphasizing whole foods such as fruits, vegetables,

Lean proteins, healthy fats, and whole grains can support overall health and provide the necessary nutrients for optimal functioning.

Hydration and Electrolyte Balance:
Adequate hydration is crucial during fasting periods, especially for women over 50 who may be more susceptible to dehydration. Drinking plenty of water and consuming electrolyte-rich beverages such as herbal teas or electrolyte-enhanced water can help maintain hydration and support electrolyte balance during fasting.

Mindful Eating Practices:
Practicing mindful eating during eating windows can help women over 50 fully appreciate and enjoy their meals while promoting better digestion and nutrient absorption. Slowing down, savoring each bite, and paying attention to hunger and fullness cues can prevent overeating and promote satisfaction from meals.

Regular Physical Activity:
Incorporating regular physical activity into daily routine complements the benefits of intermittent fasting for women over 50. Engaging in a combination of aerobic exercise, strength training, and flexibility exercises can support overall health, muscle maintenance, bone density, and metabolic function.

Monitoring Health Metrics:
Women over 50 should monitor key health metrics such as weight, blood pressure, blood sugar levels, cholesterol levels, and markers of inflammation regularly. Tracking changes in health parameters can help assess the impact of intermittent fasting on overall health and make any necessary adjustments to the fasting regimen.

By adhering to these principles, women over 50 can implement intermittent fasting in a safe, effective, and sustainable manner, harnessing its potential benefits to optimize health and wellbeing during this stage of life.

CHAPTER TWO

Hormones and Menopause

Intermittent fasting (IF) has gained popularity for its potential health benefits, particularly among women over 50 who are navigating the challenges of hormonal changes associated with menopause. Understanding how intermittent fasting impacts hormones during this stage of life is crucial for optimizing health and well-being.

Estrogen and Progesterone Decline: Menopause brings about a significant decline in estrogen and progesterone levels, leading to various symptoms such as hot flashes, mood swings, and weight gain. Intermittent fasting may offer some relief by improving insulin sensitivity and promoting fat loss, which can help mitigate these symptoms.

Insulin Sensitivity: Insulin resistance often increases with age and hormonal changes, contributing to weight gain and metabolic disturbances. Intermittent fasting has been shown to enhance insulin sensitivity, potentially reducing the risk of insulin-related conditions like type 2 diabetes and metabolic syndrome in menopausal women.

Growth Hormone: Intermittent fasting can stimulate the production of growth hormone, which plays a crucial role in metabolism, muscle maintenance, and fat loss. This can be particularly beneficial for women over 50, as declining growth hormone levels are associated with decreased muscle mass and increased fat accumulation.

Cortisol Regulation: Chronic stress and hormonal fluctuations during menopause can dysregulate cortisol levels, leading to increased abdominal fat and heightened inflammation. Intermittent fasting, when practiced correctly and without excessive stress, may help regulate cortisol levels and reduce the negative impact of stress on the body.

Thyroid Function: Some women experience changes in thyroid function during menopause, which can affect metabolism and energy levels. While intermittent fasting has been shown to have mixed effects on thyroid hormones, it's essential for women over 50 to monitor their thyroid health and adjust their fasting protocol accordingly.

Bone Health: Estrogen decline during menopause increases the risk of osteoporosis and bone fractures. Intermittent fasting, when combined with a balanced diet rich in calcium and vitamin D, may support bone health by promoting the production of osteocalcin, a hormone involved in bone formation.

Menopausal Symptoms: While intermittent fasting may offer metabolic benefits for women over 50, it's essential to consider individual differences and potential impacts on menopausal symptoms. Some women may find that fasting exacerbates hot flashes or disrupts sleep patterns, while others may experience improvements in mood and energy levels.

In summary, intermittent fasting has the potential to impact hormone levels in women over 50, which may provide metabolic and health benefits during the menopause. However, women should proceed cautiously when fasting, taking into account their unique health status, hormone levels, and menopausal symptoms. It is recommended that women seek advice from a healthcare provider or nutritionist prior to beginning any fasting regimen, especially at this stage of life.

Understanding Hormonal Changes During Menopause

Menopause, a natural biological process, marks the end of a woman's reproductive years and is characterized by significant hormonal changes. Understanding how menopause affects hormones is crucial for women over 50 considering intermittent fasting as part of their health regimen.

Estrogen Decline: One of the primary hormonal changes during menopause is the decline in estrogen production by the ovaries. Estrogen plays a crucial role in regulating the menstrual cycle, maintaining bone density, and supporting various bodily functions. The decrease in estrogen levels during menopause can lead to symptoms such as hot flashes, night sweats, vaginal dryness, and mood swings.

Progesterone Decline: Progesterone is important in regulating the menstrual cycle and promoting pregnancy; its reduction can lead to irregular menstrual cycles and worsen symptoms like mood swings and sleeplessness in certain women. Progesterone levels fall throughout menopause along with estrogen.

Impact on Metabolism: Estrogen decline during menopause can also affect metabolism. Women may experience a decrease in metabolic rate and an increase in abdominal fat deposition. These changes can contribute to weight gain, insulin resistance, and an increased risk of metabolic disorders such as type 2 diabetes and cardiovascular disease.

Insulin Sensitivity: Hormonal changes during menopause can affect insulin sensitivity, leading to fluctuations in blood sugar levels. Insulin resistance may increase, making it more challenging for the body to regulate glucose effectively. Intermittent fasting has been shown to improve insulin sensitivity, potentially helping to mitigate these metabolic changes associated with menopause.

Thyroid Function: Menopause can also impact thyroid function in some women. Thyroid hormones play a crucial role in metabolism, energy regulation, and overall well-being. Some women may experience changes in thyroid hormone levels during menopause, which can affect metabolism and energy levels. It's essential to monitor thyroid health when considering intermittent fasting, as fasting may influence thyroid function in susceptible individuals.

Bone Health: Estrogen decline during menopause increases the risk of osteoporosis and bone fractures. Estrogen plays a vital role in maintaining bone density by inhibiting bone resorption. As estrogen levels decline, bone loss accelerates, leading to an increased risk of fractures. Intermittent fasting, when combined with a nutrient-rich diet, exercise, and adequate calcium and vitamin D intake, may help support bone health during menopause.

Consultation and Monitoring: Before embarking on an intermittent fasting regimen, especially during menopause, women should consult with a healthcare provider or nutritionist. Monitoring hormone levels, metabolic parameters, and overall well-being is essential to ensure that intermittent fasting is safe and appropriate for individual health needs and goals.

In summary, women over 50 who are thinking about intermittent fasting must comprehend the hormonal changes that come with menopause. Even though the menopause causes major hormonal changes that may affect bone health, metabolism, and general well-being, intermittent fasting may be able to help manage these changes. To guarantee safety and efficacy, intermittent fasting must be done carefully and under the supervision of a specialist, especially during this life-transitional stage.

How Intermittent Fasting Affects Hormones

A nutritional strategy called intermittent fasting (IF) alternates between periods of eating and fasting. Due to its possible health advantages, including effects on hormones, it has become more popular. Here's a thorough examination of the hormonal effects of intermittent fasting:

Insulin: Intermittent fasting can lead to improved insulin sensitivity, which is the body's ability to respond to insulin and regulate blood sugar levels effectively. During fasting periods, insulin levels decrease, allowing the body to use stored glucose for energy. Over time, this can help lower fasting blood sugar levels and reduce the risk of insulin resistance, type 2 diabetes, and metabolic syndrome.

Growth Hormone (GH): Intermittent fasting has been shown to increase the secretion of growth hormone, especially during fasting periods. Growth hormone plays a crucial role in metabolism, muscle growth, fat burning, and overall health. Higher levels of growth hormone promote fat loss, preserve muscle mass, and support cellular repair and regeneration.

Norepinephrine and Epinephrine: Intermittent fasting can stimulate the release of norepinephrine and epinephrine, also known as noradrenaline and adrenaline, respectively. These hormones increase alertness, focus, and energy expenditure. Elevated levels of norepinephrine and epinephrine during fasting periods help mobilize stored energy (fat) for fuel, leading to increased fat burning and weight loss.

Cortisol: Cortisol is a stress hormone that plays a role in metabolism, inflammation, and stress response. While intermittent fasting can temporarily increase cortisol levels during fasting periods, chronic stress and prolonged fasting may lead to dysregulation of cortisol levels. It's essential to practice intermittent fasting in a way that minimizes stress and supports overall well-being.

Leptin and Ghrelin: Intermittent fasting can affect hunger and satiety hormones, such as leptin and ghrelin. Leptin, produced by fat cells, signals fullness and helps regulate energy balance. Ghrelin, produced by the stomach, signals hunger and stimulates appetite. Some studies suggest that intermittent fasting may lead to changes in leptin and ghrelin levels, resulting in reduced appetite and improved hunger control.

Thyroid Hormones: Intermittent fasting may affect thyroid hormone levels, including triiodothyronine (T3) and thyroxine (T4), which regulate metabolism, energy production, and body temperature. While short-term intermittent fasting typically does not have a significant impact on thyroid function in healthy individuals, prolonged fasting or excessive calorie restriction may lead to changes in thyroid hormone levels. It's essential to monitor thyroid health and adjust fasting protocols accordingly, especially for individuals with thyroid conditions.

In summary, intermittent fasting affects various hormones in the body, influencing metabolism, fat burning, appetite regulation, and overall health. When practiced correctly and in moderation, intermittent fasting can promote hormonal balance, metabolic flexibility, and weight management. However, it's essential to consider individual differences, health status, and goals when incorporating intermittent fasting into a lifestyle regimen. Consulting with a healthcare provider or nutritionist can help ensure that intermittent fasting is safe and suitable for individual needs.

Managing Menopause Symptoms with Intermittent Fasting

Menopause, a natural stage in a woman's life, brings about hormonal changes that can lead to various symptoms, including hot flashes, mood swings, weight gain, and sleep disturbances. Intermittent fasting (IF) has emerged as a potential strategy for managing some of these menopausal symptoms. Here's how intermittent fasting can help alleviate menopause symptoms in women over 50:

Improved Insulin Sensitivity: Insulin resistance often increases with age and hormonal changes, contributing to weight gain and metabolic disturbances during menopause. It has been demonstrated that intermittent fasting increases insulin sensitivity, enabling the body to more effectively control blood sugar levels. By enhancing insulin sensitivity, intermittent fasting may help stabilize energy levels and reduce the risk of insulin-related conditions like type 2 diabetes, which can exacerbate menopausal symptoms.

Weight Management: Many women experience weight gain during menopause, particularly around the abdomen. Intermittent fasting can be an effective strategy for managing weight during this stage of life. By restricting the timing of food intake and promoting fat loss, intermittent fasting may help women over 50 maintain a healthy weight and reduce the risk of obesity-related health issues, such as cardiovascular disease and joint problems.

Hormonal Balance: Intermittent fasting may influence hormone levels in women over 50, potentially offering relief from menopausal symptoms. While more research is needed in this area, some studies suggest that intermittent fasting could help regulate hormone levels, including estrogen and progesterone, which decline during menopause. By promoting hormonal balance, intermittent fasting may alleviate symptoms such as hot flashes, mood swings, and sleep disturbances.

Reduced Inflammation: Chronic inflammation is believed to play a role in the development and severity of menopausal symptoms.It has been demonstrated that intermittent fasting lowers pro-inflammatory marker levels, which in turn reduces inflammation in the body. By reducing inflammation, intermittent fasting may help alleviate symptoms such as joint pain, headaches, and fatigue commonly associated with menopause.

Enhanced Mood and Mental Health: Mood swings, irritability, and anxiety are common during menopause due to hormonal fluctuations. Intermittent fasting has been shown to have mood-enhancing effects by promoting the release of neurotransmitters like serotonin and dopamine. By improving mood and mental well-being, intermittent fasting may help women over 50 cope with the emotional challenges of menopause and maintain a positive outlook on life.

Consultation and Monitoring: Before starting an intermittent fasting regimen to manage menopause symptoms, women over 50 should consult with a healthcare provider or nutritionist. Monitoring overall health, hormone levels, and symptom severity is essential to ensure that intermittent fasting is safe and effective for individual needs and goals. Additionally, it's important to approach intermittent fasting gradually and listen to the body's signals to avoid excessive stress or negative side effects.

In summary, intermittent fasting shows promise as a potential strategy for managing menopause symptoms in women over 50. By improving insulin sensitivity, promoting weight management, balancing hormones, reducing inflammation, and enhancing mood and mental health, intermittent fasting may offer relief from common menopausal symptoms. However, it's crucial for women to approach intermittent fasting with caution, seek professional guidance, and listen to their bodies to ensure safety and effectiveness during this transformative stage of life.

CHAPTER THREE

Getting Started with Intermittent Fasting

Getting started with intermittent fasting (IF) involves understanding the concept and gradually incorporating it into your lifestyle. Here's a comprehensive guide:

Understand Intermittent Fasting: IF is an eating pattern that cycles between periods of fasting and eating.It suggests when to consume certain foods rather than which ones to eat in particular.

Choose Your Method: There are several methods of IF. Some popular ones include:
16/8 Method: 16 hours of fasting followed by an 8-hour window for meals each day.
5:2 Diet: Eating normally for 5 days a week and restricting calorie intake to 500-600 calories for 2 non-consecutive days.

Eat-Stop-Eat: Fasting for 24 hours once or twice a week.

Alternate-Day Fasting: A eating pattern that alternates between days of abundance and days of abstinence.

Consult Your Doctor: Before starting IF, especially if you have any underlying health conditions or concerns, it's advisable to consult with your healthcare provider.
Start Slowly: If you're new to fasting, start with a less restrictive method like the 16/8 method and gradually increase fasting periods as you become accustomed to it.

Keep Hydrated: To stay hydrated and help suppress hunger, drink lots of water when fasting.

Choose Nutrient-Dense Foods: During eating windows, focus on consuming whole, nutrient-dense foods to fuel your body properly.

Listen to Your Body: Pay attention to how you feel during fasting periods. If you experience extreme hunger, dizziness, or other discomfort, adjust your fasting schedule accordingly.

Be Flexible: IF doesn't have to be rigid. If your schedule or circumstances change, it's okay to adapt your fasting window accordingly.

Monitor Progress: Keep track of your progress, including weight loss, energy levels, and overall well-being, to see if IF is working for you.

Combine with Exercise: Regular exercise can complement intermittent fasting by enhancing its benefits. Just ensure to fuel your workouts appropriately during eating windows.

Be Patient: Results may not be immediate. Give your body time to adjust to the new eating pattern and be patient with yourself throughout the process.

Remember, intermittent fasting isn't suitable for everyone, and it's essential to find an approach that works for your individual lifestyle and health needs.

Finding the Right Fasting Schedule

When choosing a fasting schedule, women over 50 should take their overall health, metabolism, and hormonal changes into account. Here's a thorough guide:

See Your Doctor: It's important to speak with your doctor before beginning any fasting regimen, particularly if you're over 50. They are able to evaluate your condition and make tailored advice.

Recognize Hormonal Changes: Women over 50 undergo hormonal changes, especially after menopause, which can impact hunger signals and metabolism. Comprehending these modifications might assist in customizing a fasting regimen that suits your body the finest.

Think about Metabolism: As we age, our metabolism slows down, which makes maintaining a healthy weight more difficult. The fasting schedule should be modified in accordance with the benefits of intermittent fasting, which include increased metabolism and weight loss.

Start Gradually: As your body adjusts, start with a less stringent fasting plan and progressively extend the fasting intervals. Start with a 12-hour fast, for instance, then work your way up to 14 or 16 hours if that's more comfortable.

Pick a Sustainable Method: Decide on an intermittent fasting strategy that fits your tastes and way of life. Strategies like the 16/8 method—which involves fasting for 16 hours and eating within an 8-hour window—or the 5:2 diet—which involves eating regularly for 5 days and limiting calories for 2 days—might be appropriate.

Pay Attention to Your Body: Observe your body's reaction to the fast. You should think about changing your fasting schedule or technique if you suffer from excessive hunger, exhaustion, or other negative effects.

Take into Account Your Nutrient Needs: As you become older, it's critical to make sure you're getting enough calcium and vitamin D for strong bones. During eating windows, include nutrient-dense foods in your meals.

Keep Yourself Hydrated: To stay hydrated and reduce hunger during the fasting time, drink lots of water. During fasting periods, you can also drink black coffee and herbal teas, but stay away from sugary or high-calorie drinks.

Keep an eye on health indicators: Monitor vital signs such as blood pressure, cholesterol, and sugar and/or blood pressure. See your doctor if you detect any worrying changes.

Be Adaptable: Allow yourself to modify your fasting regimen as necessary in response to your body's reactions and evolving situations. Long-term sustainability and enjoyment of a fasting regimen are crucial.

Make health and wellbeing your first priority.
Intermittent fasting is only one part of a balanced
lifestyle. Make regular exercise, social interactions,
stress reduction, and enough sleep your top
priorities to promote your general health and
well-being.

Women over 50 should be patient, try several
fasting schedules, and pay attention to their own
needs and preferences while choosing one. You can
create a fasting regimen that supports health and
vitality at this stage of life by collaborating closely
with your healthcare professional and paying
attention to your body.

Popular Intermittent Fasting Protocols

Popular intermittent fasting protocols include various methods that cycle between periods of eating and fasting. Here's a comprehensive overview:

The 16/8 Method (Restricted Eating by Time):
Fasting Period: A 16-hour fast is observed every day.
Eating Window: Eat every meal throughout a period of eight hours.
For instance, eat your meals between 12 and 8 p.m. and forgo breakfast.

5:2 Diet:
Fasting Period: Eat normally for 5 days of the week.
Restriction Period: Limit calorie intake to 500-600 calories on 2 non-consecutive days.
Example: Eat normally from Monday to Friday and restrict calories on Wednesday and Saturday.

Eat-Stop-Eat:

Fasting Period: Fast for 24 hours once or twice a week.

Example: Fast from dinner one day until dinner the next day, or from breakfast to breakfast.

Alternate-Day Fasting:
Fasting Period: Alternate between days of regular eating and fasting.
Example: Eat normally on Monday, fast on Tuesday, eat normally on Wednesday, and so on.

OMAD (One Meal A Day):
Fasting Period: Fast for approximately 23 hours each day.
Eating Window: Consume all daily calories within a one-hour window.
Example: Eat one large meal at dinner time and fast for the rest of the day.

Warrior Diet:
Fasting Period: Fast for 20 hours each day.
Eating Window: Consume all meals within a 4-hour window, typically in the evening.
Example: Fast throughout the day and eat one large meal in the evening, followed by a smaller meal.

24-Hour Fast:
Fasting Period: Fast for a full 24-hour period, once or twice a week.
Example: Fast from dinner one day to dinner the next day.

36-Hour Fast:
Fasting Period: Extend fasting to a full 36 hours, once or twice a week.
Example: Fast from dinner one day until breakfast two days later.

These guidelines can be modified to fit specific tastes, way of life, and health objectives. Selecting a fasting technique that works for you is important, and speaking with a healthcare provider is advised—especially if you have any underlying medical issues or concerns. Moreover, while observing intermittent fasting, maintaining hydration and having nutrient-dense meals throughout eating windows might enhance general health and wellbeing.

Adapting Fasting to Your Way of Life

As we age, our bodies undergo natural changes that can affect our metabolism, energy levels, and overall health. Intermittent fasting can be a great way to take control of our well-being, but it's essential to adapt it to our unique needs and lifestyle.

Here's the thing: intermittent fasting isn't a one-size-fits-all approach. As women over 50, we need to consider our hormonal changes, menopause symptoms, and other health factors when starting a fasting regimen.

So, how can we make intermittent fasting work for us?

- **Start slow**: Begin with shorter fasting windows (12-14 hours) and gradually increase as your body adjusts.

- **Listen to your body**: If you're feeling weak, dizzy, or experiencing other negative side effects, it's okay to slow down or modify your fasting schedule.

- **Prioritize nutrient-dense foods**: Focus on whole, nutrient-rich foods during your eating windows to support your overall health.
- **Stay hydrated**: Drink plenty of water during fasting periods to help reduce hunger and support detoxification.
- **Be mindful of hormones**: If you're experiencing menopause symptoms, consider adjusting your fasting schedule to accommodate your hormonal fluctuations.
- **Consult a healthcare professional**: Before starting any new fasting regimen, consult with your healthcare provider to ensure it's safe and suitable for your individual needs.

Remember, intermittent fasting is a personal journey, and it's crucial to adapt it to your unique needs and lifestyle. By being mindful of our bodies and making adjustments as needed, we can enjoy the benefits of intermittent fasting while prioritizing our overall health and well-being.

Preparing for Your Fasting Journey

Well done on taking the initial step toward beginning your experience of intermittent fasting! We understand that changing isn't always simple, but as women over 50, we're here to encourage and mentor you every step of the way.

Let's get ready before you start! The following advice will assist you in positioning yourself for success:

1. **Speak with your doctor**: It's crucial to speak with your healthcare practitioner before beginning any new diet or fasting regimen, particularly if you have any underlying medical concerns.

2. **Recognize your objectives**: State your motivation for attempting intermittent fasting. Is it to lower inflammation, increase energy, or decrease

weight? Being mindful of your targets will sustain your motivation.

3. **Get knowledge of various techniques**: Find the intermittent fasting strategy that works best for you by researching different approaches, such as 16:8, 5:2, or Eat-Stop-Eat.

4. **Arrange your fasting schedule:** Pick a timetable that works for your social obligations and way of living. If necessary, you might need to change the days or windows when you fast.

5. Stock up on full, nutrient-dense foods like fruits, vegetables, lean proteins, and healthy fats. Throw out processed and high-sugar meals.

6. **Remain hydrated:** To aid with detoxifying and lessen hunger, drink lots of water prior to, during, and following fasting times.

7. **Remember to treat yourself with kindness:** It's acceptable to go slowly and make adjustments as

necessary. If you make a mistake, don't be too hard on yourself; just get back on course.

8. **Find support**: Find a friend to travel with or join a community. Having assistance has a significant impact!

9. **Pay attention to your body**: Modify your fasting schedule based on your hunger and fullness cues.

10. **Have patience**: Results from intermittent fasting can take some time to manifest. It's a journey. Prioritize development above perfection!

You'll be well-equipped to begin your intermittent fasting quest and position yourself for success if you pay attention to these pointers.

Mental Preparation

Intermittent fasting has become quite popular, and you might be considering it to manage your health, weight, or energy levels. For women over 50, it can be a helpful tool, but it's important to approach it with a clear and positive mindset. Here are a few tips on how to mentally prepare for intermittent fasting at this stage of life.

1. Understand Your Why
Start by getting clear on why you want to try intermittent fasting. Is it to lose weight, boost energy, or manage a health condition? When you understand your reasons, it's easier to stay committed. Write down your goals and keep them somewhere you can see them every day.

2. Learn About Fasting

Before diving in, take some time to learn about intermittent fasting. There are different approaches, like the 16/8 method or the 5:2 plan. Research what might work best for you and your lifestyle. Being prepared for what's ahead alleviates anxiety and doubt.

3. Set Realistic Expectations

Intermittent fasting isn't a magic bullet, and it might take some time to see results. As your body adjusts, experiencing ups and downs is typical. Be consistent at all times and set reasonable expectations. Setbacks are normal; just keep going forward.

4. Plan Your Schedule

Create a fasting schedule that fits your life. If you're used to having breakfast every morning, it might take some adjustment. You can start with shorter fasting windows and gradually increase them as you get comfortable. Having a plan helps you stay on track and reduces anxiety about the unknown.

5. Find Support

Doing intermittent fasting alone can be challenging. Find a friend or a group to join you, or look for online communities where you can share experiences and get advice. Realizing you have company can be a powerful driving force.

6. **Be Kind to Yourself**

Remember, your body and mind are unique. If you have a day where fasting feels too difficult, it's okay to adjust or take a break. Observe your body and treat yourself with kindness. It's about growth, not about perfection.

7. **Focus on Health, Not Just Weight**

While intermittent fasting can lead to weight loss, it's not the only benefit. Focus on how you feel—your energy levels, sleep quality, and mood. These are just as important as any number on a scale.

8. **Stay Hydrated and Nourished**

During your eating windows, make sure you're getting enough nutrients and staying hydrated.

Eating a balanced diet and drinking plenty of water will help you feel good and stay energized.

9. Consult a Professional
If you have any health concerns or existing conditions, it's a good idea to talk to a doctor or a nutritionist before starting intermittent fasting. They can assist you in developing a strategy that works well and is safe for you.

With these mental preparation tips, you can approach intermittent fasting with a positive mindset and a sense of readiness. Take it one step at a time, and remember that your journey is unique to you.

Setting Realistic Expectations

Intermittent fasting has gained a lot of popularity for its potential health benefits, but it's important to set realistic expectations, especially for women over 50. Let's talk about what you can expect and some key things to keep in mind as you consider intermittent fasting.

What to Expect from Intermittent Fasting
Intermittent fasting can be an effective approach for managing weight, improving metabolic health, and even enhancing mental clarity. However, it's not a magic bullet, and results can vary from person to person. Here's what you might experience:

- **Weight Loss**: Many people try intermittent fasting for weight loss, and while it can be effective, it's not guaranteed. You may see gradual changes in your weight, but they might not be dramatic or immediate. It's essential to pair intermittent fasting with a balanced diet and regular exercise for best results.

- **Energy Levels**: Some people report increased energy and focus during fasting periods, but others may feel sluggish or lightheaded. If you find that fasting impacts your energy levels negatively, you may need to adjust the fasting schedule or duration to suit your body's needs.
- **Menopausal Considerations**: For women over 50, hormonal changes can affect how intermittent fasting works. You might experience shifts in appetite, metabolism, or even mood. It's critical to listen to your body and make adjustments as needed.

Tips for Success

To make intermittent fasting work for you, consider these tips:

- **Choose a Suitable Fasting Schedule**: There are many fasting schedules, from 16/8 to 5:2. Experiment to find one that fits your lifestyle and makes you feel good. It's okay to try different approaches to see what suits you best.

- **Prioritize Nutrition**: Fasting isn't just about skipping meals. When you do eat, focus on nutrient-dense foods like vegetables, fruits, lean proteins, and whole grains. This will help maintain your energy and support overall health.

- **Stay Hydrated:** Water is your friend during fasting periods. Staying hydrated helps curb hunger and keeps you feeling your best.

- **Consult Your Doctor**: If you have underlying health conditions or are taking medication, talk to your doctor before starting intermittent fasting. They can help you determine if it's safe and suggest modifications if needed.

Be Patient with Yourself

Fasting intermittently is a journey rather than a race. It's critical to practice self-compassion and patience. You may support your health and well-being in a variety of ways if you decide it's not the right fit. Finding what works for you and helps you feel your best is ultimately what matters.

CHAPTER FOUR

Intermittent Fasting Methods for Women over 50

If you're a woman over 50 and thinking about trying intermittent fasting, you've probably heard a lot about its potential benefits for weight management, energy, and overall health. But with all the different fasting methods out there, it's easy to feel overwhelmed. Let's break it down and talk about a few popular intermittent fasting methods that might work well for you.

The 16/8 Method

This is one of the most straightforward intermittent fasting methods. You fast for 16 hours and then eat during an 8-hour window. Many people find this schedule manageable because it often means skipping breakfast and having two meals during the day. For example, you might eat from noon to 8 p.m. This approach gives your body a good break without feeling too restrictive.

The 5:2 Diet

With the 5:2 diet, you eat normally for five days of the week, and on two non-consecutive days, you limit your calorie intake to around 500-600 calories. This method can be a great way to start intermittent fasting if you're not ready to fast every day. It's flexible, and you can choose the fasting days that best fit your schedule.

The Alternate-Day Fasting Method

As the name suggests, this method involves fasting every other day. On fasting days, you might consume a very low-calorie meal or fast entirely, and on non-fasting days, you eat normally. This method can be more intense, but some women find it helpful for weight loss or breaking through a plateau.

The Eat-Stop-Eat Method

This approach involves abstaining from food for a complete day, either weekly or every other week. For example, you might eat dinner at 7 p.m. and not eat again until 7 p.m. the next day. This approach can be a bit challenging, but it can also help reset your eating habits and give your body a longer break from food.

Tips for Success with Intermittent Fasting

Whichever method you choose, here are a few tips to help you succeed:

- **Start Slowly**: If you're new to intermittent fasting, start with a shorter fasting window and gradually increase it as you get more comfortable. There's no rush.
- **Hydrate adequately**: Drink plenty of water throughout fasting periods to stay replenished. Herbal teas and black coffee are also good options if you want something with a bit of flavor.

- **Eat Nutrient-Dense Foods**: When you're in your eating window, focus on foods that are rich in nutrients—think vegetables, lean proteins, whole grains, and healthy fats. You'll feel content and invigorated doing this.
- **Listen to Your Body**: If you're feeling dizzy, overly tired, or experiencing other discomforts, don't hesitate to adjust your fasting schedule. Intermittent fasting should support your health, not compromise it.
- **Consult with a Professional**: Before you start any new fasting regimen, especially as a woman over 50, it's a good idea to check

with a healthcare professional or a registered dietitian. They can offer personalized advice and help you navigate any potential health risks.

Intermittent fasting can be a great way to improve your health, but it's important to find the method that works best for you. Try out different approaches and see what feels right. Remember, it's all about creating a sustainable routine that makes you feel good. Good luck, and remember to be kind to yourself as you explore this journey.

Time-Restricted Eating

Intermittent fasting (IF) has gained popularity for its potential health benefits, and time-restricted eating is a common approach that many women over 50 find both practical and effective. If you're considering intermittent fasting and want a simple way to start, time-restricted eating could be just what you're looking for.

What Is Time-Restricted Eating?

Time-restricted eating is a type of intermittent fasting where you limit your eating to a specific window of time each day. For example, you might eat only between 12 p.m. and 8 p.m., creating a 16-hour fasting period overnight. This approach doesn't require you to count calories or follow a strict meal plan—it's more about when you eat rather than what you eat.

Why Time-Restricted Eating?
For women over 50, this method can be appealing because it's flexible and easy to fit into a busy lifestyle. It also aligns with the body's natural rhythms, allowing you to eat during the day and fast at night when you're likely to be asleep.

Time-restricted eating has been linked to several benefits, including:

- **Weight Management**: By limiting your eating window, you might naturally consume fewer calories, which can help with weight loss or maintenance.

- **Improved Metabolism**: Fasting periods give your body a break from constant digestion, which can improve metabolic health.Better Insulin Sensitivity: This can be especially beneficial as women age, helping to reduce the risk of type 2 diabetes.
- **Reduced Inflammation**: Some studies suggest that intermittent fasting can reduce inflammation, which is linked to various health issues.

Tips for Getting Started

If you're interested in time-restricted eating, here are some tips to help you get started and make it work for you:

- **Choose Your Eating Window**: Decide on a window that fits your lifestyle. Common choices are 16/8, where you fast for 16 hours and eat during an 8-hour window, or 14/10, which gives you a 10-hour eating window. Start with what feels manageable.

- **Ease Into It**: If you're new to intermittent fasting, don't feel like you have to jump into a long fasting period right away. Start with a 12-hour fast and gradually increase it as you get comfortable.
- **Stay Hydrated**: During your fasting period, drink plenty of water. Herbal teas and black coffee are also fine, as long as they don't contain added sugars or cream. Staying hydrated helps curb hunger and keeps you feeling refreshed.

- **Eat Nutritious Foods**: When you're in your eating window, focus on whole, nutrient-dense foods. Include plenty of vegetables, lean proteins, whole grains, and healthy fats to keep you energized and satisfied.
- **Listen to Your Body**: If you experience dizziness, fatigue, or other discomforts, it's okay to adjust your fasting schedule. Time-restricted eating should enhance your health, not make you feel worse.

- **Consult a Healthcare Professional:** If you have underlying health conditions or concerns about fasting, it's always a good idea to consult a healthcare professional or a registered dietitian before starting. Their guidance is customized to meet your specific health needs.

16/8 Method

If you're a woman over 50 considering intermittent fasting, the 16/8 method might be a good place to start. This approach is popular because it's straightforward and can fit into almost any lifestyle. Let's break it down and talk about how it works, why it's a good choice, and how you can get started.

What Is the 16/8 Method?

The 16/8 method involves fasting for 16 hours and then eating during an 8-hour window each day. It might sound like a long time to go without eating, but remember that a lot of those fasting hours are while you're asleep. So, if you finish dinner at 7 p.m., you wouldn't eat again until 11 a.m. the next day. This way, you're just skipping breakfast and having lunch and dinner as usual.

Why the 16/8 Method for Women Over 50?

For women over 50, the 16/8 method has some great advantages. It can help with weight management, improve metabolic health, and even boost energy levels. Here's why it stands out as an excellent option:

- **Simplicity**: You don't need to count calories or follow a complicated meal plan. Just stick to your eating window and fast for 16 hours.

- **Adaptability**: Adjust the eating window to suit your busy schedule. If you're a morning person, you might eat from 9am to 5pm If you're a night owl, you could eat from noon to 8 p.m.
- **Improved Metabolism**: Fasting for 16 hours gives your body a break from constant digestion, which can help improve metabolism and support weight loss or maintenance.

- **Potential Health Benefits**: Some studies suggest intermittent fasting can improve insulin sensitivity, reduce inflammation, and even promote heart health.

Getting Started with the 16/8 Method

Ready to give it a try? Here are some tips to help you get started with the 16/8 method:

- **Choose Your Eating Window**: Decide on an 8-hour window that fits your daily routine. It might take a bit of trial and error to find what works best, but that's okay.
- **Ease Into It:** If 16 hours of fasting feels daunting, start with a shorter fasting period and gradually increase it. You might start with a 12-hour fast and work your way up to 16 hours.
- **Stay Hydrated**: During the fasting period, make sure you're drinking plenty of water. Herbal teas and black coffee (without sugar or cream) are also fine and can help you stay hydrated.

- **Focus on Nutrition**: When you're in your eating window, prioritize nutrient-dense foods like vegetables, lean proteins, whole grains, and healthy fats. This will help you feel full and satisfied.
- **Listen to Your Body**: Pay attention to how you feel during the fasting period. If you're feeling dizzy, overly tired, or uncomfortable, consider adjusting your fasting schedule or taking a break.

- **Get Support**: Having a friend or joining an online community of people doing intermittent fasting can be helpful. It's always nice to share experiences and get tips from others.
- **Consult a Healthcare Professional:** If you have any underlying health conditions or concerns, it's a good idea to talk to a healthcare professional or registered dietitian before starting intermittent fasting. They can give you personalized advice to ensure it's safe for you.

Final Thoughts

The 16/8 method can be a simple and effective way to try intermittent fasting, especially for women over 50. It's flexible, easy to follow, and has the potential to bring several health benefits. Start slow, be kind to yourself, and find the eating window that works best for you. Good luck, and here's to a healthier, more energized you!

14/10 Method

What is the 14/10 Method and How Does It Work?

The 14/10 Method is a type of intermittent fasting where you fast for 14 hours and then eat within a 10-hour window. For example, you might eat from 8am to 6pm, fasting from 6 p.m. until 8 a.m. the next morning. The objective is to grant your body a temporary reprieve from constant food intake, enabling it to recover and recalibrate.

Benefits of the 14/10 Method

Here are some of the key benefits of the 14/10 Method:

- **Weight Loss:** By limiting the eating window, you may consume fewer calories, leading to weight loss.
- **Improved Insulin Sensitivity**: Fasting can help your body become more sensitive to insulin, reducing the risk of diabetes.
- **Increased Human Growth Hormone Production:** Some studies suggest that fasting can boost the production of human growth hormone (HGH), which helps with muscle growth and fat loss.
- **Digestive Health**: Giving your digestive system a break can improve gut health and reduce inflammation.

How to Implement the 14/10 Method

Starting the 14/10 Method is simple but may require some adjustments to your eating schedule. To get you going, consider these pointers:

- **Choose Your Eating Window**: Pick a 10-hour window that works for you. If you're a morning person, start early; if you prefer eating later, start later.
- **Gradual Adjustment**: If 14 hours of fasting seems too long, start with a shorter fasting period and gradually increase it.
- **Stay Hydrated**: Drink plenty of water during the fasting period to stay hydrated and manage hunger.

- **Plan Meals**: Plan your meals to ensure you get a balanced diet within your eating window.
- **Avoid Late-Night Eating**: Try to avoid eating just before bedtime to allow your body to rest.

Common Challenges and How to Overcome Them

While the 14/10 Method is generally straightforward, you might encounter some challenges:
- **Hunger**: If you find yourself feeling hungry during the fasting period, try drinking water or herbal tea to curb the craving.
- **Social Events**: If your eating window conflicts with social events, plan ahead by eating before or adjusting your window for that day.
- **Consistency**: Sticking to a schedule can be challenging. Set reminders or use a fasting app to help you stay on track.

Comparison with Other Intermittent Fasting Methods

The 14/10 Method is just one of many intermittent fasting approaches. Here's how it compares with other popular methods:

- **16/8 Method**: This approach involves a 16-hour fasting window and an 8-hour eating window. It's a bit stricter than the 14/10 Method but may lead to faster results.
- **5:2 Diet**: This method involves eating normally for five days and reducing calorie intake to about 500-600 calories for two non-consecutive days. It's more flexible but might be harder to stick to.
- **Alternate Day Fasting**: In this approach, you fast every other day, eating normally on the alternating days. This method requires more discipline and might not suit everyone.

Final Thoughts

The 14/10 Method is a sustainable and effective approach to healthy eating and weight management. It offers flexibility and allows you to choose an eating window that fits your lifestyle. If you're looking to improve your health and potentially lose weight, this method could be a great starting point.

Before starting any fasting method, it's essential to consult with a healthcare professional, especially if you have underlying health conditions or take medication. With the right approach and mindset, the 14/10 Method can be a valuable tool in your health journey. Good luck, and happy fasting!

Alternate-Day Fasting

Alternate-Day Fasting is one technique that many women over 50 find intriguing. Alternate-day fasting has become popular as a means of weight loss and better health. This approach is precisely what it sounds like: you fast for one day and then resume regular eating the following day.

Here's how it works. On your fasting days, you can still have a small number of calories—typically around 500—but the idea is to keep it very light. Some people stick to broth, tea, or small portions of fruits and vegetables. The key is to give your body a break from heavy meals and let it focus on other things, like healing and repairing.

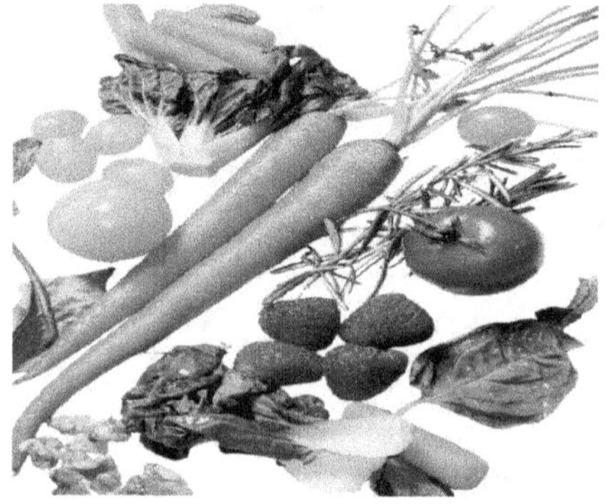

On your eating days, you're free to eat your usual meals, but it's still a good idea to choose nutritious foods and avoid overdoing it. It's not a free pass to binge; instead, it's about finding a balanced approach to eating that feels sustainable.

Why do women over 50 find this approach appealing? Well, for starters, it's flexible. You don't have to restrict yourself every day, which can be tough for some. With alternate-day fasting, you can plan your eating days around social events, family dinners, or when you know you might need extra energy.

There are also some health benefits that might be particularly relevant for women over 50. Research suggests that intermittent fasting can help improve metabolic health, reduce inflammation, and even support brain health. And because it's relatively simple, it can be easier to stick with than more complicated diets.

However, it's important to remember that intermittent fasting isn't for everyone. If you have certain health conditions or take medications that require food, you'll need to talk to your doctor before trying this approach. And if you ever feel unwell during fasting, it's crucial to listen to your body and adjust as needed.

In the end, Alternate-Day Fasting can be a helpful tool for women over 50 looking to manage their weight and improve their health. It's flexible, straightforward, and can be tailored to fit your lifestyle. Just be sure to approach it with an open mind, and remember that the goal is to find what works best for you.

Modified Alternate-Day Fasting

In recent years, intermittent fasting (IF) has become increasingly popular as a means to enhance overall health, achieve weight loss, and potentially extend lifespan. This eating pattern involves alternating between periods of consumption and abstinence, with various methods to choose from. Specifically, women over 50 have shown interest in Modified Alternate-Day Fasting (MADF), a balanced approach that incorporates fasting into a healthy lifestyle without extreme restrictions. This method offers a sustainable and manageable way to reap the benefits of intermittent fasting while maintaining overall well-being.

What is Modified Alternate-Day Fasting?

Modified Alternate-Day Fasting is a type of intermittent fasting where you alternate between days of reduced calorie intake and days of normal eating. Unlike strict alternate-day fasting, which requires a complete fast or very low-calorie intake on fasting days, MADF allows for a moderate

amount of calories, usually about 500–600, on the fasting days. This approach provides flexibility while still offering the benefits of intermittent fasting.

Why is it Popular Among Women Over 50?

Women over 50 often experience unique health challenges, including hormonal changes, menopause-related symptoms, reduced metabolism, and an increased risk of chronic diseases. Modified Alternate-Day Fasting can be particularly appealing for this age group for several reasons:

- **Simplicity**: MADF is easy to follow because it doesn't require complex meal planning or strict calorie counting on eating days. This simplicity can make it more sustainable over the long term.
- **Flexibility:** The modified approach allows some food intake on fasting days, which can be helpful for women who are concerned about energy levels, especially those who are physically active or have busy schedules.

- **Health Benefits**: Intermittent fasting, including Modified Alternate Day Fasting, has been associated with various health benefits. For women over 50, these benefits might include improved heart health, better blood sugar control, reduced inflammation, and potential weight loss. There's also evidence suggesting that intermittent fasting can support brain health, which is important as women age.

- **Reduced Hormonal Stress:** Complete fasting can stress the body, potentially affecting hormones like cortisol and insulin. By allowing a moderate calorie intake on fasting days, Modified Alternate Day Fasting may reduce the risk of hormonal imbalances, making it a safer option for women dealing with menopause-related changes.

How to Get Started with Modified Alternate-Day Fasting

If you're interested in trying Modified Alternate Day Fasting, here are some tips to help you get started:

- **Consult a Healthcare Professional**: Before starting any fasting regimen, it's important to consult with a healthcare provider, especially if you have underlying health conditions or are taking medication.
- **Choose Your Fasting Days**: With Modified Alternate Day Fasting, you'll need to decide which days will be your fasting days. Many people choose non-consecutive days, such as Monday, Wednesday, and Friday, but find what works best for your schedule.
- **Plan Your Fasting Day Meals**: On fasting days, aim for about 500–600 calories. Include foods that are high in protein and fiber to help you feel full. Soups, salads, and small portions of lean protein are good choices.

- **Keep Yourself Hydrated**: To stay hydrated, sip lots of water throughout the day. Black coffee and herbal teas are also excellent choices.
- **Pay Attention to Your Body:** Observe your body's reaction to the fast. If you feel

lightheaded, extremely tired, or have other unsettling symptoms, change the days you fast or see a doctor.

5:2 Method

The 5:2 method is one of the most straightforward approaches to intermittent fasting, offering a balance between flexibility and structure. In this guide, we'll dive into what the 5:2 method is, why it might work for women over 50, and how to get started.

What Is the 5:2 Method?

The 5:2 method involves eating normally for five days of the week and then significantly restricting calories on the other two non-consecutive days. On the fasting days, women typically consume about 500–600 calories, while the other days are just like any regular eating day. This pattern creates a manageable way to practice intermittent fasting without feeling overly restricted.

Why Is It a Good Fit for Women Over 50?

Women over 50 face unique health changes due to menopause, shifting hormones, and a slower metabolism. Here's why the 5:2 method can be a good fit for this age group:

- **Flexibility**: With five days of normal eating, it's easier to enjoy social gatherings, family meals, and special occasions without worrying about sticking to a strict diet. The flexibility makes it less likely that you'll feel deprived or frustrated.
- **Simple Structure**: The 5:2 method is easy to understand and implement. You don't have to count calories or track every bite on the normal eating days. This simplicity can be a relief for women who don't want the stress of complex diet plans.
- **Health Benefits:** Intermittent fasting, including the 5:2 method, has been linked to several health benefits. For women over 50, it can help with weight loss or maintenance, improve insulin sensitivity, and potentially lower the risk of chronic diseases like diabetes and heart disease.
- **Reduced Stress on the Body**: By allowing a moderate intake on fasting days, the 5:2 method is less likely to cause extreme hunger or fatigue. This can be important for women who are already experiencing

hormonal fluctuations and other changes in energy levels.

How to Start with the 5:2 Method

If you're curious about trying the 5:2 method, here are some steps to help you get started:

- **Pick Your Fasting Days:** Choose two non-consecutive days for your reduced-calorie intake. Many people select Mondays and Thursdays, but you can choose any days that fit your schedule.
- **Plan Your Meals for Fasting Days**: Aim for 500–600 calories on fasting days. Consider small meals or snacks that are high in protein and fiber, like eggs, low-fat yogurt, vegetables, and fruit.

- **Stay Hydrated**: Drink plenty of water, herbal tea, or black coffee to stay hydrated and curb hunger on fasting days.
- **Don't Overcompensate on Normal Days:** The idea of the 5:2 method is to maintain a balanced eating pattern. On your regular

eating days, try not to overeat and maintain a nutritious diet rich in whole foods and well-balanced nutrients.

- **Listen to Your Body**: Everyone's experience with fasting is different. If you feel lightheaded, excessively hungry, or unwell, it's okay to adjust the fasting days or the amount of calories you consume. Always prioritize your health and well-being.

Final Thoughts

The 5:2 method is a flexible and straightforward way to practice intermittent fasting, making it ideal for women over 50. It allows you to maintain a normal eating routine while still reaping the benefits of fasting. If you're considering trying it, be sure to listen to your body, make adjustments as needed, and enjoy the journey to better health.

Extended Fasting

The practice of intermittent fasting, or IF, has grown in popularity as a way to control weight and enhance general health. There are several approaches to choose from, and it entails times of fasting and restricted food. One such technique is extended fasting, which usually entails a fast of longer than twenty-four hours. Extended fasting may seem intimidating to women over 50, but with the right support and attention, it can be a useful tool to help achieve certain health objectives.

What is Extended Fasting?

Extended fasting refers to fasting for longer periods, generally more than 24 hours, and can stretch to several days. While some approaches to intermittent fasting focus on shorter periods of fasting each day, extended fasting is more intense and requires careful planning and consideration.

Why Might Extended Fasting Appeal to Women Over 50?

Women over 50 experience a range of physiological changes, from menopause to a slower metabolism, that can affect health and weight. Extended fasting might appeal to some women in this age group for a variety of reasons:

- **Health Reset**: Extended fasting can give the body a break from constant food intake, potentially leading to improvements in digestion, energy levels, and inflammation. Some believe that fasting can help "reset" the body, giving it a chance to cleanse and rejuvenate.
- **Potential Weight Loss**: For women struggling with weight gain, especially during or after menopause, extended fasting can lead to significant calorie reduction, contributing to weight loss over time. It may also help kick-start metabolism in some cases.
- **Autophagy and Cellular Health**: Extended fasting is associated with autophagy, a process where the body cleans out damaged cells and regenerates new ones. This could be beneficial for women over 50 seeking

ways to support longevity and cellular health.

- **Mental Clarity and Focus**: Some people report improved focus and mental clarity during extended fasting. This can be helpful for women juggling work, family, and personal commitments.

Things to Consider Before Trying Extended Fasting

Extended fasting isn't for everyone. It's crucial to understand the potential risks and prepare properly. Here are a few things to consider:

- **Consult with a Healthcare Professional:** Before attempting extended fasting, especially for periods longer than 24 hours, it's crucial to consult with a healthcare provider. They can help you assess whether it's safe for you and suggest precautions to take.

- **Hydration is Key**: Staying hydrated is essential during extended fasting. Drink plenty of water, herbal teas, or electrolyte-rich beverages to prevent dehydration.

- **Ease Into It:** If you're new to intermittent fasting, it's best to start with shorter fasting periods and gradually increase them. Jumping into extended fasting without preparation can be tough on the body.
- **Monitor Your Body's Response**: Pay attention to how your body reacts to extended fasting. If you experience dizziness, extreme fatigue, nausea, or any other concerning symptoms, it's important to break the fast and seek medical advice.
- **Break the Fast Slowly:** After an extended fast, reintroduce food slowly and in small portions to avoid overwhelming your digestive system.

Benefits and Risks

For women over 50, intermittent fasting can offer unique advantages, but it's also important to understand the risks. Let's break down the benefits and risks of intermittent fasting for women over 50 in a way that's easy to understand.

Benefits of sporadic Fasting for Women Over 50

Many people turn to intermittent fasting for its potential health benefits. Here are some of the key reasons women over 50 might find it appealing:

- **Weight Loss and Management**: Menopause and hormonal changes can make weight loss a challenge for women over 50. Intermittent fasting can help reduce calorie intake and boost metabolism, which can lead to weight loss or easier weight management.
- **Improved Insulin Sensitivity**: IF has been linked to improved insulin sensitivity, which can be especially important as women age and become more prone to insulin resistance and type 2 diabetes.

- **Reduced Inflammation**: Some studies suggest that intermittent fasting can reduce inflammation in the body. This can be beneficial for women over 50 who may be at higher risk for inflammatory conditions like arthritis or heart disease.
- **Heart Health:** Intermittent fasting might also help reduce risk factors for heart disease, such as high blood pressure and cholesterol. Given that heart disease risk increases with age, this can be a significant benefit.
- **Mental Clarity and Focus**: Some people find that intermittent fasting gives them a mental boost. If you're juggling multiple responsibilities and need to stay sharp, this could be a welcome advantage.
- **Longevity and Autophagy**: Intermittent fasting has been linked to the process of autophagy, where the body cleans out damaged cells and generates new ones. This process can support longevity and cellular health, which is particularly important as we age.

Risks of Intermittent Fasting for Women Over 50

While there are benefits to intermittent fasting, it's crucial to be aware of the potential risks, especially for women over 50. Remember to consider the following:

- **Hormonal Imbalances**: Intermittent fasting can sometimes lead to hormonal fluctuations, particularly with strict fasting patterns. For women over 50 dealing with menopause or other hormonal changes, this could exacerbate symptoms.
- **Nutrient Deficiency**: If fasting isn't balanced with proper nutrition, it could lead to deficiencies in essential vitamins and minerals. Women over 50 need to ensure they're getting enough calcium, vitamin D, and other nutrients crucial for bone health and overall well-being.
- **Energy and Fatigue:** Some people find that fasting makes them feel weak or tired, which can affect daily activities. If you lead a busy life or need steady energy throughout the day, this could be a concern.

- **Social Impact**: Intermittent fasting can impact social activities, especially if it involves meal-based gatherings. This might lead to feelings of isolation or difficulty participating in social events.
- **Medical Conditions**: If you have pre-existing medical conditions, such as diabetes, heart disease, or eating disorders, intermittent fasting might not be suitable without careful medical supervision.

CHAPTER FIVE

Nutrition and Meal Planning

As we age, our nutritional needs may change, and it becomes increasingly important to nourish our bodies with the right foods. Intermittent fasting can be a powerful tool for promoting health and well-being in women over 50, but it's important to ensure that your meals are packed with essential nutrients to support overall health.

1. **Prioritize Nutrient-Dense Foods:**

Focus on incorporating nutrient-dense foods into your meals, including:

- **Lean proteins**: such as poultry, fish, tofu, beans, and lentils, to support muscle mass and repair.
- **Fruits and vegetables**: aim for a colorful variety to provide essential vitamins, minerals, and antioxidants.

- **Whole grains:** such as brown rice, quinoa, oats, and whole wheat bread, for sustained energy and fiber.
- **Healthy fats:** found in foods like avocados, nuts, seeds, and olive oil, to support heart health and brain function.
- **Dairy or dairy alternatives:** for calcium and vitamin D to support bone health.

2. Balance Macros:

Ensure that your meals are balanced with the right mix of macronutrients:

- **Protein**: aim to include a source of protein in each meal to support muscle maintenance and repair.
- **Carbohydrates:** choose complex carbohydrates to provide sustained energy and fiber to keep you feeling full.
- **Fats:** incorporate healthy fats into your meals for satiety and to support hormone production and nutrient absorption.

3. **Hydration**:

Drink plenty of water, herbal teas, and other non-caloric drinks to stay hydrated throughout the day. In addition to being beneficial for general health, hydration helps reduce hunger when fasting.

4. **Meal Timing**:

Plan your meals to coincide with your eating window during intermittent fasting. Focus on spreading your meals evenly throughout the day to ensure adequate energy intake and to prevent overeating during your eating window.

5. **Snack Smart**:

If you find yourself getting hungry between meals, opt for nutrient-dense snacks such as fruits, vegetables with hummus, Greek yogurt, or nuts. These snacks can help tide you over until your next meal without derailing your fasting efforts.

6. **Consult a Healthcare Professional:**
If you have any underlying health conditions or
specific dietary needs, it's essential to consult with a
healthcare professional or registered dietitian before
starting intermittent fasting. They can provide
personalized guidance and ensure that you're
meeting your nutritional requirements.

In summary, meal preparation and nutrition are
critical for maintaining the health and wellbeing of
women over 50 who engage in intermittent fasting.
You may maximize the advantages of intermittent
fasting for general health and vitality by
concentrating on nutrient-dense foods, balancing
macros, drinking enough water, and speaking with a
healthcare provider.

Nutritional Guidelines for Women over 50

Women's nutritional demands vary with age. Women go through menopause after the age of 50, which can result in a variety of hormonal and physical changes. For women in this age range, intermittent fasting (IF) can be a healthy eating pattern; however, in order to maintain maximum health, it is imperative to adhere to appropriate dietary standards. The following are detailed dietary recommendations for women over 50 who follow intermittent fasting:

1. **Protein**: Aim for 1.2-1.6 grams of protein per kilogram of body weight from sources like lean meats, fish, eggs, tofu, legumes, and dairy. Protein helps maintain muscle mass and bone density.

2. **Calcium:** Ensure adequate calcium intake (1,200 mg/day) from sources like dairy, leafy greens, and fortified plant-based milk to support bone health.

3. **Vitamin D:** Maintain sufficient vitamin D levels (600-800 IU/day) through sun exposure, supplements, or fortified foods to support bone health and immune function.

4. **Omega-3 fatty acids**: Include sources like fatty fish, flaxseeds, and walnuts in your diet to support heart health and brain function.

5. **Fiber**: Aim for 25-30 grams of fiber per day from whole foods like fruits, vegetables, whole grains, and legumes to support digestive health and satiety.

6. **Hydration**: Drink plenty of water (at least 8 cups/day) and limit sugary drinks.

7. **Whole foods**: Focus on whole, unprocessed foods, and limit packaged and processed foods.

8. **Healthy fats**: Include sources like avocado, nuts, and seeds in your diet to support heart health and satiety.

9. **Vitamin B12**: Ensure adequate vitamin B12 intake (2.4 mcg/day) from animal sources or supplements to support energy production and nerve function.

10. **Iron**: Maintain sufficient iron levels (8 mg/day) from sources like lean meats, beans, and fortified cereals to support healthy red blood cells.

11. **Zinc**: Include zinc-rich foods like oysters, beef, and chicken in your diet to support immune function and wound healing.

12. **Potassium**: Aim for 4,700 mg/day from sources like bananas, leafy greens, and sweet potatoes to support heart health and blood pressure management.

13. **Vitamin K:** Ensure adequate vitamin K intake (90 mcg/day) from leafy greens and fermented foods to support bone health and blood clotting.

14. **Magnesium**: Maintain sufficient magnesium levels (320 mg/day) from sources like dark leafy greens, nuts, and whole grains to support muscle and nerve function.

15. **Probiotics**: Include probiotic-rich foods like yogurt, kefir, and fermented vegetables in your diet to support gut health and immune function.

When practicing IF, consider the following:

- Eat nutrient-dense foods during your eating windows.
- Avoid excessive sugar and saturated fat intake.
- Stay hydrated during fasting periods.
- Pay attention to your body and modify your plan as necessary.
- To develop a customized plan, speak with a certified dietitian or healthcare professional.

Essential Nutrients

Women's nutritional demands vary with age, so it's critical to make sure they're obtaining the nutrients they need to maintain general health and wellbeing, particularly during intermittent fasting. Women over 50 should pay particular attention to these important nutrients:

1. Protein:

Protein is essential for maintaining muscle mass, supporting immune function, and repairing tissues. As women age, they may need slightly more protein to support muscle maintenance and repair. Lean meats, poultry, fish, eggs, dairy products, legumes, tofu, and tempeh are all excellent sources of protein.

2. Calcium and Vitamin D:

Calcium and vitamin D are crucial for maintaining bone health and preventing osteoporosis, a condition that becomes more prevalent in women over 50. Dairy products, fortified plant-based milk alternatives,

Leafy green vegetables, tofu, and almonds are good sources of calcium. Vitamin D can be obtained from sunlight exposure and fortified foods such as fatty fish, egg yolks, and fortified dairy or plant-based milk.

3. Omega-3 Fatty Acids:
Omega-3 fatty acids are important for heart health, brain function, and reducing inflammation. Fatty fish like salmon, mackerel, and sardines are excellent sources of omega-3s. Walnuts, hemp seeds, chia seeds, and flaxseeds are examples of plant-based sources.

4. Fiber:
Fiber is essential for digestive health, maintaining regular bowel movements, and controlling blood sugar levels. Women over 50 should aim to consume plenty of fiber-rich foods such as fruits, vegetables, whole grains, legumes, nuts, and seeds.

5. **B Vitamins:**

B vitamins are essential for neuron function, energy metabolism, and red blood cell formation. Foods rich in B vitamins include whole grains, leafy green vegetables, legumes, nuts, seeds, eggs, poultry, fish, and dairy products.

6. **Magnesium:**

Magnesium is involved in over 300 biochemical reactions in the body and is essential for bone health, muscle function, and nerve function. Good sources of magnesium include leafy green vegetables, whole grains, nuts, seeds, legumes, and dark chocolate.

7. **Potassium:**

Potassium is important for maintaining fluid balance, muscle contractions, and heart function. Foods high in potassium include bananas, oranges, potatoes, sweet potatoes, avocados, leafy green vegetables, and beans.

8. **Antioxidants:**
Antioxidants help protect the body from oxidative stress and inflammation, which can contribute to age-related diseases. Colorful fruits and vegetables, berries, nuts, seeds, green tea, and dark chocolate are rich sources of antioxidants.

In summary, for women over 50 who practice intermittent fasting, it is crucial to ensure that they are getting enough of these vital nutrients. Women can enhance their general health and maximize their nutritional intake by focusing on nutrient-dense meals and adhering to a balanced diet as they age. A licensed dietician or other healthcare expert can offer individualized advice and make sure that each person's dietary needs are satisfied.

Foods to Emphasize and Avoid

Foods to Emphasize:

- **Lean Proteins**: Incorporate sources of lean protein into your meals to support muscle maintenance and repair. Examples include chicken, turkey, fish, tofu, tempeh, beans, lentils, and Greek yogurt.
- **Fruits and Vegetables**: Load up on a variety of colorful fruits and vegetables to provide essential vitamins, minerals, antioxidants, and fiber. In order to make sure you're getting a variety of nutrients, aim for a rainbow of colors.
- **Whole Grains**: Choose whole grains over refined grains to provide sustained energy and fiber to keep you feeling full. Opt for options like brown rice, quinoa, oats, barley, whole wheat bread, and whole grain pasta.

- **Healthy Fats**: Include sources of healthy fats in your diet to support heart health, brain function, and hormone production. Examples include avocados, nuts, seeds, olive oil, fatty fish (such as salmon, mackerel, and sardines), and coconut oil.
- **Dairy or Dairy Alternatives**: Incorporate dairy products or dairy alternatives fortified with calcium and vitamin D to support bone health. Choose options like milk, yogurt, cheese, and fortified plant-based milk alternatives.
- **Hydration:** Stay hydrated throughout the day by drinking lots of water, particularly during fasting. For hydration without breaking your fast, you can also consume herbal teas, infused water, and sparkling water.

Foods to Avoid:

- **Processed Foods**: Minimize your intake of processed foods high in added sugars, unhealthy fats, and preservatives. These include sugary snacks, baked goods, fast food, processed meats, and sugary beverages.
- **Refined Grains**: Limit your consumption of refined grains like white bread, white rice, and sugary cereals, as they can cause spikes in blood sugar levels and lead to energy crashes.
- **Highly Processed Snacks**: Avoid highly processed snacks like chips, crackers, and candy, as they are often high in unhealthy fats, sugars, and sodium. Instead, opt for whole food snacks like nuts, seeds, fruit, and veggies with hummus.
- **Excessive Alcohol**: While moderate alcohol consumption may be acceptable for some, excessive alcohol intake can disrupt sleep, impair metabolism, and contribute to weight gain. Limit alcohol consumption and opt for healthier alternatives like herbal tea or sparkling water.

- **Unhealthy Fats:** Limit your intake of unhealthy fats like trans fats and saturated fats, which can increase the risk of heart disease. Avoid foods like fried foods, processed meats, and high-fat dairy products.
- **Sugary Beverages**: Steer clear of sugary beverages like soda, fruit juice, and sweetened coffee drinks, as they can contribute to weight gain and increase the risk of chronic diseases like type 2 diabetes and heart disease.

Women over 50 can promote their health and well-being while intermittent fasting by emphasizing nutrient-dense foods and avoiding processed and harmful options. Always pay attention to your body's signals of hunger and fullness, and for individualized advice and assistance, speak with a medical practitioner or registered dietitian.

Balanced Meals for Fasting and Feeding Windows

Intermittent fasting can be an effective way for women over 50 to manage their weight and improve overall health. To make the most of fasting and feeding windows, it's important to focus on creating balanced meals that provide essential nutrients and support satiety. Here's how to do it:

1. Fasting Window Meals:

During the fasting window, it's essential to avoid consuming calories. However, you can still include non-caloric beverages like water, herbal tea, and black coffee to help curb hunger and stay hydrated.

2. Feeding Window Meals:

When it's time to eat, aim to create balanced meals that include a mix of protein, carbohydrates, and healthy fats to provide sustained energy and keep you feeling full. Here's a breakdown of what to include in your feeding window meals:

- **Protein**: Incorporate a source of lean protein into each meal to support muscle maintenance and repair. Good options include poultry, fish, tofu, tempeh, beans, lentils, and Greek yogurt.
- **Carbohydrates**: Choose complex carbohydrates to provide energy and fiber to keep you feeling full. Opt for whole grains like brown rice, quinoa, oats, and whole wheat bread, as well as fruits and vegetables.
- **Healthy Fats**: Include sources of healthy fats to support heart health and promote satiety. Examples include avocados, nuts, seeds, olive oil, and fatty fish like salmon.
- **Vegetables**: Make vegetables a key component of your meals to provide essential vitamins, minerals, and antioxidants. Aim to fill half of your plate with non-starchy vegetables like leafy greens, broccoli, cauliflower, peppers, and carrots.

- **Hydration**: Don't forget to drink plenty of water throughout the day, especially during your feeding window, to stay hydrated and support overall health.

3. Sample Balanced Meals:

Here are some examples of balanced meals that you can enjoy during your feeding window:

- Grilled chicken breast with quinoa, roasted vegetables (such as broccoli and carrots), and a side salad with mixed greens, tomatoes, cucumbers, and balsamic vinaigrette.
- Baked salmon with sweet potato wedges, steamed asparagus, and a side of mixed berries for dessert.
- Stir-fried tofu with brown rice, stir-fried vegetables (such as bell peppers, snap peas, and mushrooms), and a sprinkle of sesame seeds for added crunch.
- Greek yogurt parfait with Greek yogurt, fresh fruit (such as berries or sliced banana), and a handful of nuts or seeds for added protein and crunch.

4. **Listen to Your Body:**
Remember to listen to your body's hunger and
fullness cues during both fasting and feeding
windows. Eat until you feel satisfied, but not overly
full, and pay attention to how different foods make
you feel.

By focusing on balanced meals that provide
essential nutrients and support satiety, women over
50 can make the most of intermittent fasting for
improved health and well-being. Experiment with
different meal combinations and find what works
best for you and your lifestyle.

Healthy Snack Ideas

Snacking can be a great way to fuel your body and keep hunger at bay during intermittent fasting. Here are some nutritious and satisfying snack options to consider:

Greek Yogurt with Berries: Greek yogurt is rich in protein, which can help keep you feeling full, while berries provide antioxidants and fiber. Mix plain Greek yogurt with fresh berries like strawberries, blueberries, or raspberries for a delicious and nutritious snack.

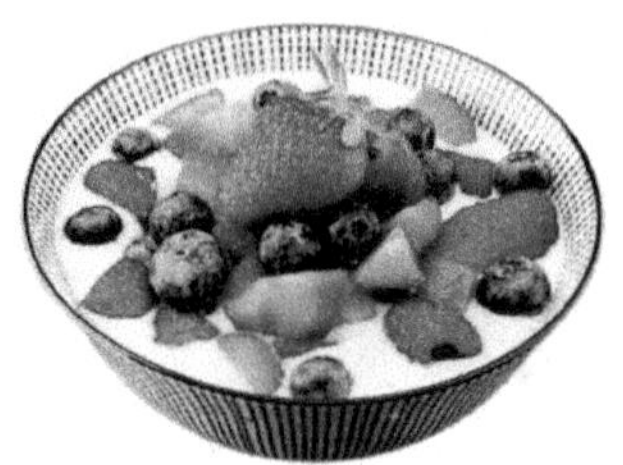

Greek Yogurt with Berries

Nuts and Seeds: Nuts and seeds are packed with healthy fats, protein, and fiber, making them an excellent choice for a satisfying snack. Choose varieties like almonds, walnuts, pumpkin seeds, or sunflower seeds, and enjoy them on their own or mixed with dried fruit for a sweet and savory combination.

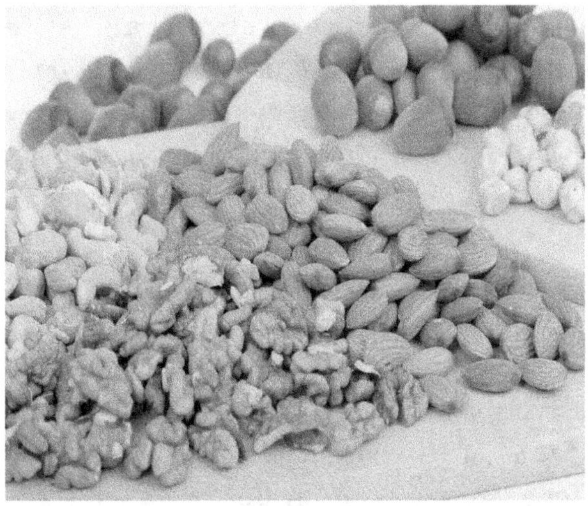

Nuts and Seeds

Vegetable Sticks with Hummus: Crisp, crunchy vegetable sticks paired with creamy hummus make for a nutritious and satisfying snack. Try dipping carrot sticks, celery, cucumber slices, bell pepper strips, or cherry tomatoes into your favorite flavor of hummus for a tasty treat.

Hard-Boiled Eggs: Hard-boiled eggs are a convenient and portable snack that provides a good source of protein and essential nutrients like vitamins D and B12. Enjoy a hard-boiled egg on its own or sliced over whole grain crackers for extra fiber.

Cottage Cheese with Fruit: Cottage cheese is high in protein and low in fat, making it a great option for a satisfying snack. Top cottage cheese with your favorite fruits, such as pineapple, peaches, or mango, for a sweet and creamy treat.

Edamame: Edamame, or steamed soybeans, are a nutritious and protein-rich snack that's perfect for munching on during the day. Simply steam frozen edamame according to package instructions, sprinkle with a little sea salt, and enjoy them warm or chilled.

Avocado Toast: Avocado toast is a delicious and nutritious snack that's easy to make and customize. Spread mashed avocado on whole grain toast and top with sliced tomatoes, a sprinkle of sea salt, and a drizzle of olive oil for a satisfying snack packed with healthy fats and fiber.

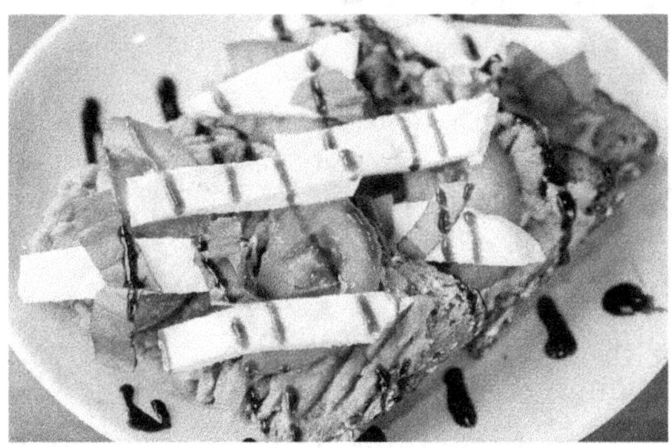

Avocado Toast

Roasted Chickpeas: Packed with protein and fiber, roasted chickpeas are a crunchy, tasty snack. Toss cooked chickpeas with olive oil, sea salt, and your favorite seasonings, such as garlic powder, paprika, or cumin, then roast them in the oven until crispy.

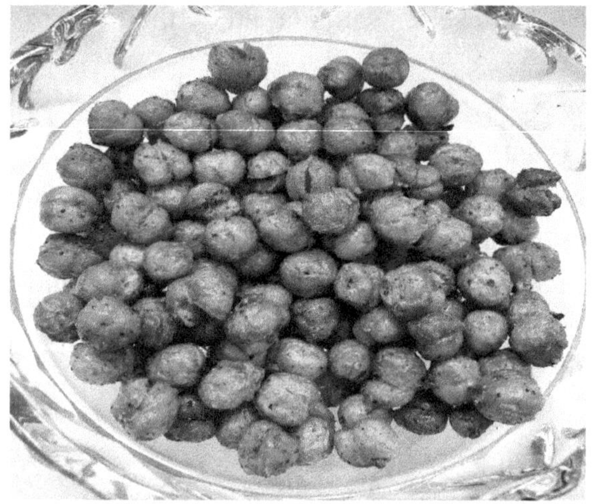

Roasted Chickpeas

To stay full and energized throughout the day, pay attention to your body's hunger cues and select snacks that offer a balance of protein, healthy fats, and fiber. As you incorporate these wholesome snack ideas into your intermittent fasting regimen, enjoy!

CHAPTER SIX

Managing Potential Challenges

For women over 50, intermittent fasting has many health advantages, such as better metabolic health, weight control, and enhanced energy. It may, however, present a unique set of difficulties, just like any nutritional strategy. Through comprehension and resolution of these obstacles, women above 50 years of age can enhance their experience with intermittent fasting. Here's how to handle possible difficulties:

Hunger and Cravings:
Solution: Stay hydrated by drinking plenty of water, herbal tea, and black coffee during fasting periods. Consuming fiber-rich foods and incorporating healthy fats and proteins into meals can also help increase satiety and reduce hunger.

Energy Levels:

Solution: Prioritize nutrient-dense foods during eating windows to provide sustained energy. Include complex carbohydrates, lean proteins, healthy fats, and plenty of fruits and vegetables in your meals to fuel your body effectively.

Nutrient Deficiencies:

Solution: Focus on consuming a variety of nutrient-dense foods to ensure you're meeting your nutritional needs. Consider incorporating supplements if necessary, especially for nutrients like vitamin D, calcium, and B vitamins, which may be deficient in some populations.

Social Situations:

Solution: Plan ahead for social events by adjusting your fasting schedule or making mindful choices about what and when to eat. Focus on enjoying the company of others rather than solely focusing on food, and don't be afraid to communicate your dietary preferences and goals to friends and family.

Exercise Performance:
Solution: Adjust your exercise routine as needed to accommodate fasting periods. Consider scheduling workouts during feeding windows when energy levels are higher, and listen to your body's signals to avoid overexertion.

Sleep Quality:
Solution: Pay attention to your sleep hygiene practices, such as establishing a regular sleep schedule, creating a comfortable sleep environment, and practicing relaxation techniques before bed. Avoid consuming caffeine or large meals close to bedtime, as they may disrupt sleep.

Digestive Issues:
Solution: Increase your intake of fiber-rich foods like fruits, vegetables, whole grains, and legumes to support digestive health. Stay hydrated and consider incorporating fermented foods like yogurt, kefir, and sauerkraut, which contain beneficial probiotics.

Plateaus or Weight Regain:
Solution: Monitor your progress and adjust your fasting schedule or meal plan as needed to break through plateaus. Focus on making sustainable lifestyle changes rather than relying solely on intermittent fasting for weight management.

By proactively addressing these potential challenges, women over 50 can navigate intermittent fasting with greater ease and maximize its benefits for their health and well-being. Remember to listen to your body, prioritize self-care, and seek support from healthcare professionals or registered dietitians as needed.

Dealing with Hunger and Cravings

Hunger and cravings are common challenges that women over 50 may face when practicing intermittent fasting. However, there are strategies to help manage these sensations and stay on track with your fasting goals. Here's how to deal with hunger and cravings:

Keep Yourself Hydrated: Throughout the day, sipping water can help suppress appetite and keep you feeling satisfied. To stay hydrated and lessen hunger pangs during fasting times, choose black coffee, herbal tea, or water.

Consume Fiber-Rich Foods: Incorporate fiber-rich foods into your meals to promote feelings of fullness and satiety. Choose fruits, vegetables, whole grains, legumes, and nuts, which can help keep you satisfied between meals.

Include Protein in Meals: Protein is known for its ability to keep you feeling full and satisfied for longer periods. Include lean sources of protein such as poultry, fish, tofu, eggs, and Greek yogurt in your meals to help reduce hunger and cravings.

Option for Healthy Fats: Healthy fats can also help curb hunger and cravings by providing a source of sustained energy. Include sources of healthy fats such as avocados, nuts, seeds, olive oil, and fatty fish in your meals and snacks.

Engage in Mindful Eating: Be aware of your body's signals of hunger and fullness when engaging in mindful eating. During meals, take your time, chew your food well, and enjoy every bite. This can lessen cravings and assist avoid overindulging.

Distract Yourself: When cravings strike, find ways to distract yourself and shift your focus away from food. Engage in activities you enjoy, such as reading, gardening, going for a walk, or practicing a hobby, to help take your mind off of food.

Plan Balanced Meals: Ensure that your meals during feeding windows are balanced and nutrient-dense, with a mix of protein, carbohydrates, and healthy fats. This can help stabilize blood sugar levels and prevent sudden spikes and crashes in hunger.

Allow for Flexibility: It's okay to occasionally indulge in your favorite foods in moderation. Allow yourself the occasional treat without guilt, but aim to maintain balance and moderation in your overall eating patterns.

Seek Support: Connect with friends, family, or online communities for support and encouragement. Sharing your experiences with others who are also practicing intermittent fasting can help you stay motivated and accountable.

Mindful Eating Techniques

Mindful eating is a powerful practice that can enhance the experience of intermittent fasting for women over 50. By being present and attentive during meals, women can cultivate a deeper connection with their food, improve digestion, and make more conscious choices about what and how they eat. Here are some comprehensive mindful eating techniques:

Pause Before Eating: Before you begin your meal, take a moment to pause and check in with yourself. Notice any sensations of hunger or fullness, as well as any emotions or thoughts that may be present.

Engage Your Senses: Make sure to use all of your senses when preparing and eating your food. Take note of the food's flavors, textures, and colors. Chew each bite slowly and deliberately, giving yourself time to enjoy the flavors and textures.

Eat Without Distractions: Minimize distractions during meals by turning off the TV, putting away your phone, and focusing solely on the act of eating. This allows you to fully experience your food and tune in to your body's hunger and fullness signals.

Practice Gratitude: Cultivate an attitude of gratitude towards your food and the process of eating. Take a moment to acknowledge the effort that went into growing, preparing, and serving your meal, and express gratitude for the nourishment it provides.

Pay Attention to Your Body: Throughout the meal, pay attention to your body's signals of hunger and fullness. Instead of stopping when your plate is empty or you feel like it, take your time eating and end when you are content.

Identify Emotional Triggers: Take note of any trends or emotional triggers that can affect your eating habits. Do you eat because it's a habit, out of boredom, or stress? You may create better coping strategies and make more deliberate decisions about how you feed yourself by being aware of these triggers.

Practice Non-Judgment: Approach your eating experience with a non-judgmental attitude towards yourself and your food choices. Let go of any guilt or shame associated with eating and allow yourself to enjoy your meals without restriction.

Be Present: Bring your full attention to the present moment as you eat, letting go of worries about the past or future. By focusing on the here and now, you can fully experience the pleasure and satisfaction of eating.

Reflect on Your Experience: After you've completed your meal, pause to consider the experience. Take note of your mental, emotional, and physical well-being. Make use of this reflection to help you better understand your body's demands and to guide your food decisions going forward.

Overcoming Plateaus and Adjusting Your Approach

Any dietary or lifestyle adjustment, including intermittent fasting, is likely to cause plateaus, particularly in women over 50. When your development slows down or stops, it's critical to modify your strategy and go past these plateaus. Here's a detailed guide on how to achieve that:

1. **Evaluate Your Progress:**
Take a step back and evaluate your progress objectively. Look at factors such as weight loss, body measurements, energy levels, and overall well-being. This assessment can help you identify areas that may need adjustment.

2. **Reassess Your Goals:**
Think about reviewing your objectives and making any required adjustments. Perhaps your priorities have changed, or maybe your original objective was too ambitious. You may stay motivated and focused

by setting reasonable and attainable goals for yourself.

3. Experiment with Fasting Protocols:

If you've been fasting the same way for a time, you might want to try some other methods. This can entail adjusting the length of your fasting window, experimenting with fasting on different days, or introducing sporadic longer fasts. Discover what suits your body and way of life the best.

4. Focus on Nutrient-Dense Foods:

Pay attention to the quality of your food choices. Emphasize nutrient-dense foods such as lean proteins, fruits, vegetables, whole grains, and healthy fats. These foods provide essential nutrients while supporting overall health and satiety.

5. Incorporate Strength Training:

Include strength training exercises in your fitness routine to help build and maintain lean muscle mass. Muscle mass is metabolically active and can help increase your resting metabolic rate, leading to improved fat loss and weight management.

6. **Manage Stress Levels:**

Chronic stress can impact weight loss efforts by increasing cortisol levels and promoting fat storage, especially around the abdomen. Practice stress-reducing techniques such as meditation, deep breathing exercises, yoga, or spending time in nature to help manage stress levels effectively.

7. **Prioritize Sleep:**

Aim for adequate and restful sleep each night, as sleep deprivation can disrupt hormonal balance and metabolism, making it harder to lose weight. Create a bedtime routine, optimize your sleep environment, and prioritize sleep hygiene practices to support quality sleep.

8. **Stay Consistent and Patient:**

Recall that advancement is a gradual process and that hitting roadblocks is normal. Maintain consistency in your eating and fasting schedule, and practice self-compassion while you overcome obstacles. Have faith in the process and acknowledge small accomplishments along the way.

9. Seek Support:
Never be afraid to ask friends, family, or online communities for help. Talk about your experiences, ask for guidance, and get ideas from those who are traveling a similar path. Having a solid support network can help you stay accountable and motivated.

10. Consult with a Healthcare Professional:
If you're struggling to overcome a plateau or have concerns about your progress, consider consulting with a healthcare professional or registered dietitian. They can provide personalized guidance, identify any underlying issues, and help you develop a tailored plan for success.

When to Seek Professional Guidance

While intermittent fasting can offer numerous benefits for women over 50, there are certain situations where seeking professional guidance is advisable to ensure safety, effectiveness, and overall well-being. Here's a comprehensive guide on when to seek professional guidance for intermittent fasting:

Pre-existing Medical Conditions:
If you have pre-existing medical conditions such as diabetes, heart disease, thyroid disorders, or eating disorders, it's essential to consult with a healthcare professional before starting intermittent fasting. They can help assess the potential risks and benefits based on your individual health status and provide personalized recommendations.

Medication Use:
Certain medications may interact with intermittent fasting or require adjustments to your fasting protocol. If you're taking prescription medications, Especially those that affect blood sugar levels, blood pressure, or metabolism, consult with your healthcare provider to ensure that intermittent fasting is safe and appropriate for you.

History of Disordered Eating:
If you have a history of disordered eating patterns such as binge eating, restrictive eating, or compulsive exercise, it's important to approach intermittent fasting with caution. Consult with a registered dietitian or mental health professional who specializes in eating disorders to develop a safe and sustainable approach to fasting.

Unintended Weight Loss or Gain:
If you experience unintended weight loss or gain while practicing intermittent fasting, it's essential to seek professional guidance to determine the underlying cause. A healthcare provider or

a registered dietitian can help assess your nutritional intake, metabolic rate, and overall health status to identify any potential issues and provide appropriate recommendations.

Persistent Hunger or Discomfort:
If you experience persistent hunger, discomfort, or adverse symptoms while fasting, it's important to address these concerns with a healthcare professional. They can help identify potential triggers, adjust your fasting protocol, and provide guidance on managing hunger and cravings effectively.

Pregnancy or Breastfeeding:
Intermittent fasting is not recommended during pregnancy or breastfeeding, as it may not provide adequate nutrition for both you and your baby. If you're pregnant, planning to become pregnant, or breastfeeding, consult with your healthcare provider for personalized nutrition recommendations that support maternal and fetal health.

Age-related Concerns:
As women age, their nutritional needs and metabolic processes may change. If you're over 50 years old and considering intermittent fasting, consult with a healthcare provider or registered dietitian who specializes in geriatric nutrition to ensure that your dietary approach supports optimal health and well-being during this life stage.

Persistent Plateaus or Challenges:
If you experience persistent plateaus, challenges, or difficulties achieving your health or weight loss goals with intermittent fasting, consider seeking professional guidance. A registered dietitian or healthcare provider can help assess your current approach, identify potential barriers, and develop a personalized plan to overcome obstacles and achieve success.

CHAPTER SEVEN

Combining Intermittent Fasting with Exercise

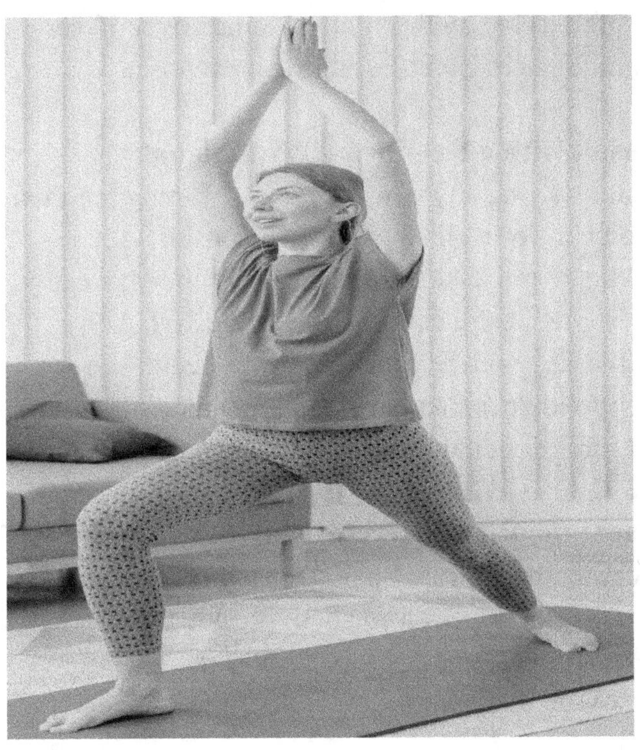

Combining intermittent fasting with exercise can be a powerful strategy for women over 50 to enhance overall health, manage weight, and improve fitness levels. However, it's essential to approach this combination thoughtfully to ensure safety, effectiveness, and optimal results. Here's a comprehensive guide on how women over 50 can combine intermittent fasting with exercise:

Consult with a Healthcare Professional:
Before starting any new exercise or fasting regimen, it's crucial for women over 50 to consult with a healthcare professional, especially if they have any underlying health conditions or concerns. A healthcare provider can assess your health status and provide personalized recommendations based on your individual needs and circumstances.

Choose the Right Exercise Routine:
Selecting the appropriate exercise routine is key for women over 50. Focus on activities that support overall fitness, strength, flexibility, and cardiovascular health.

This could include a combination of aerobic exercises (such as walking, cycling, swimming), strength training (using weights or resistance bands), and flexibility exercises (such as yoga or tai chi).

Consider Timing:
When combining intermittent fasting with exercise, consider the timing of your workouts in relation to your fasting and feeding windows. Some women may prefer to exercise during their feeding window to ensure they have enough energy and nutrients to support physical activity. Others may find that exercising during fasting periods works better for their schedule and preferences. Try out several timings to see what suits you the best.

Stay Hydrated:
Hydration is essential, especially during fasting periods and exercise. Drink plenty of water throughout the day to stay hydrated, and consider adding electrolytes if you're engaging in intense or prolonged exercise sessions. Avoid sugary sports

drinks and opt for water or electrolyte-enhanced beverages instead.

Fuel Appropriately:
If you choose to exercise during your fasting window, pay attention to your body's energy levels and fuel needs. Consuming a balanced meal or snack that includes carbohydrates, protein, and healthy fats before and/or after your workout can help support performance, recovery, and muscle maintenance.

Listen to Your Body:
Pay attention to how your body responds to exercise and fasting. If you experience dizziness, lightheadedness, weakness, or other adverse symptoms, it may indicate that you need to adjust your fasting or exercise routine. Listen to your body's signals and make modifications as needed to ensure safety and well-being.

Focus on Recovery:
Adequate rest and recovery are essential components of any exercise program, especially for women over 50. Ensure you're getting enough sleep, incorporating rest days into your routine, and

prioritizing recovery strategies such as stretching,
foam rolling, and relaxation techniques.

Track Your Progress:
Keep track of your exercise sessions, fasting
schedule, and overall progress to monitor your
results and make adjustments as needed. Tracking
can help you identify patterns, set realistic goals,
and stay motivated on your fitness journey.

By following these guidelines and listening to your
body's needs, women over 50 can effectively
combine intermittent fasting with exercise to
support their overall health and well-being.
Remember to prioritize safety, consistency, and
enjoyment in your approach, and don't hesitate to
seek guidance from a qualified healthcare
professional or fitness expert if needed.

Exercise Recommendations for Women over 50

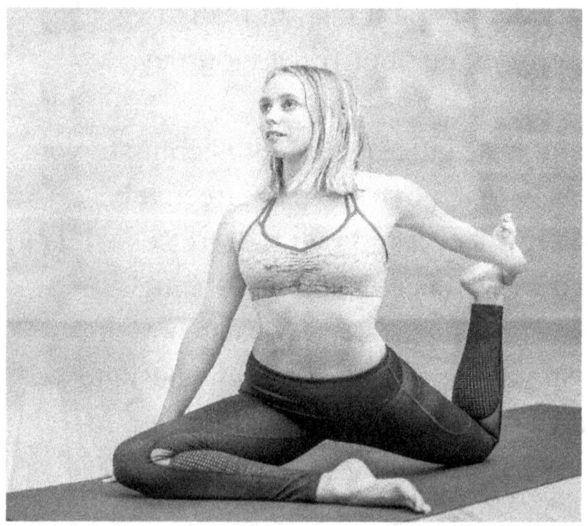

Regular exercise is important for maintaining overall health, mobility, and vitality, especially for women over 50. When combined with intermittent fasting, exercise can further enhance the benefits of this dietary approach. Here are exercise recommendations designed specifically for women over 50 practicing intermittent fasting:

Cardiovascular Exercise:

Engage in cardiovascular exercises such as walking, cycling, swimming, or dancing to improve heart health, endurance, and stamina. Try to get in at least 150 minutes a week of aerobic activity at a moderate to high level, or 75 minutes of intense activity spread out over many days.

Strength Training:

Incorporate strength training exercises into your routine to build and maintain muscle mass, which naturally declines with age. Use resistance bands, dumbbells, or bodyweight exercises to target major muscle groups such as the legs, arms, back, chest, and core. Aim for at least two days of strength training per week, with a focus on proper form and technique.

Functional Movement Training:
Incorporate functional movement exercises that mimic everyday activities to improve mobility, coordination, and functional fitness. Exercises such as squats, lunges, step-ups, and functional core exercises help build strength and stability for daily tasks like bending, lifting, and reaching.

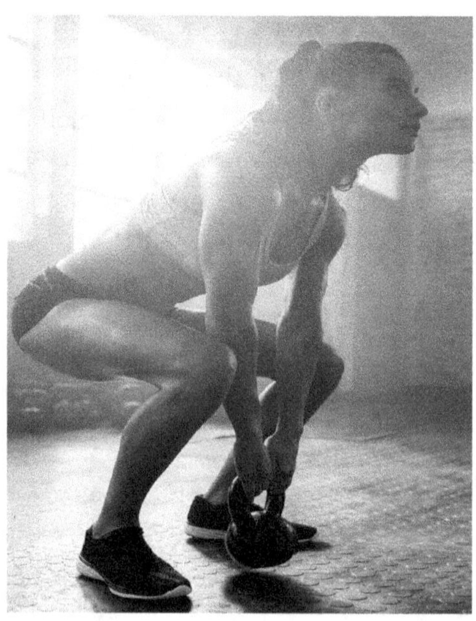

Flexibility and Balance Exercises:
Include flexibility and balance exercises to improve range of motion, joint mobility, and stability. Practices such as yoga, tai chi, or Pilates are excellent choices for enhancing flexibility, balance, and overall body awareness. Aim for sessions that focus on stretching, gentle movements, and relaxation techniques to promote flexibility and reduce the risk of injury.

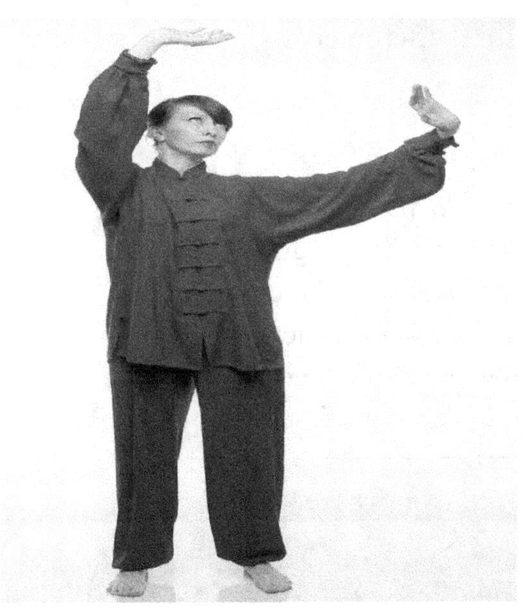

Interval Training:
Consider incorporating interval training or high-intensity interval training (HIIT) into your routine to boost calorie burn, improve cardiovascular fitness, and stimulate fat loss. Alternate between periods of high-intensity exercise and rest or low-intensity recovery to challenge your body and maximize results. As your fitness level rises, start with shorter intervals and progressively increase the time and intensity.

Mind-Body Practices:
Explore mind-body practices such as meditation, deep breathing exercises, or guided relaxation to reduce stress, enhance mental clarity, and promote overall well-being. These practices can complement your physical exercise routine and support stress management, which is especially important for women over 50.

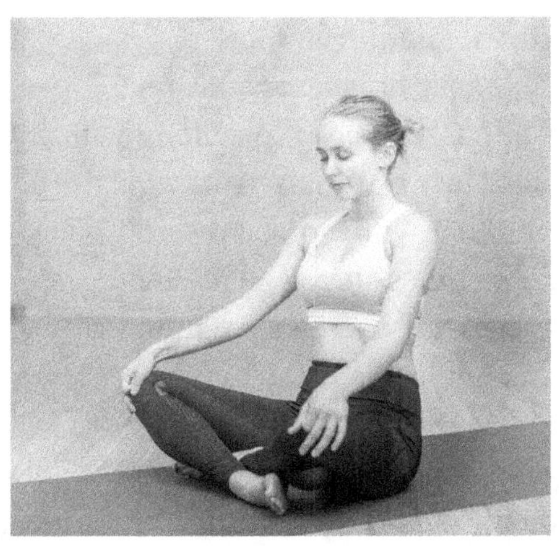

Variety and Adaptation:

Keep your exercise routine varied and adaptable to prevent boredom, plateau, and overuse injuries. Mix and match different types of exercises, vary intensity and duration, and listen to your body's cues to adjust as needed. Be open to trying new activities and exploring what works best for your body and preferences.

Consult with a Professional:

If you're new to exercise or have any health concerns or limitations, consider consulting with a certified personal trainer or fitness professional who has experience working with women over 50. They can help assess your fitness level, goals, and needs, and design a personalized exercise program that's safe, effective, and enjoyable.

You can boost general health and well-being, reap the benefits of intermittent fasting, and lead a more active and satisfying lifestyle by adhering to these workout guidelines designed specifically for women over 50. In your workout regimen, don't forget to put consistency, advancement, and fun first. Also, remember to recognize and acknowledge your success as you go.

Types of Exercise to Incorporate

For women over 50 practicing intermittent fasting, incorporating a variety of exercises into their routine is essential for overall health, fitness, and well-being. Here are several types of exercises to consider integrating into your regimen:

Cardiovascular Exercise:
Cardiovascular exercises elevate your heart rate and help improve cardiovascular health. Incorporate activities such as brisk walking, jogging, cycling, swimming, or using cardio machines like ellipticals or treadmills. Aim for at least 150 minutes of moderate-intensity aerobic activity per week.

Strength Training:
The maintenance and growth of muscle mass is facilitated by strength training, and as one ages, this is essential for maintaining bone density, metabolism, and functional independence. Incorporate movements like squats, lunges, push-ups, rows, and overhead presses that focus on

the primary muscle groups. For resistance, you can utilize machines, resistance bands, or dumbbells.

Flexibility and Mobility Work:
Flexibility and mobility exercises improve range of motion, joint health, and posture. Incorporate stretches and movements that target different muscle groups, such as yoga, Pilates, tai chi, or simple stretching routines. Focus on gentle stretches and movements to enhance flexibility without causing strain or discomfort.

Balance and Stability Training:
Balance and stability training help reduce the risk of falls and injuries, which become more prevalent with age. Include exercises that challenge balance, such as single-leg stands, heel-to-toe walks, balance board exercises, or stability ball exercises. These activities help strengthen stabilizing muscles and improve proprioception.

Functional Movement Patterns:
Functional exercises mimic movements used in daily activities and help improve overall functionality and quality of life. Examples include

squats, lunges, step-ups, bending, lifting, and reaching.

Focus on performing these movements with proper form and alignment to enhance strength, coordination, and mobility.

Interval Training:
Interval training involves alternating between periods of high-intensity exercise and rest or low-intensity recovery. This type of training can boost metabolism, improve cardiovascular fitness, and stimulate fat loss. Examples include sprint intervals, cycling sprints, or circuit training with bursts of intense effort followed by brief recovery periods.

Mind-Body Practices:
Mind-body practices promote relaxation, stress reduction, and mind-body awareness. Incorporate activities such as meditation, deep breathing exercises, progressive muscle relaxation, or guided imagery to support mental well-being and enhance the mind-body connection.

Low-Impact Exercise Options:
Low-impact exercises are gentle on the joints and suitable for individuals with joint pain, arthritis, or mobility limitations. Options include swimming, water aerobics, stationary biking, using an elliptical machine, or walking on flat surfaces. These activities provide cardiovascular benefits without putting excessive stress on the joints.

Outdoor Activities:
Take advantage of outdoor activities that combine exercise with fresh air and nature. Activities such as hiking, gardening, golfing, or outdoor yoga classes provide physical and mental health benefits while enjoying the outdoors.

Women over 50 who practice intermittent fasting can maintain their physical activity, health, and vitality by combining these different forms of exercise into their schedule. Always pick enjoyable activities, pay attention to your body's signals, and seek advice from a fitness specialist or medical professional if you have any restrictions or concerns.

Timing Exercise with Fasting Windows

Integrating exercise with intermittent fasting requires thoughtful planning, especially for women over 50. By strategically timing exercise sessions within fasting windows, women can maximize the benefits of both practices while supporting their overall health and well-being. Here's a comprehensive guide on how to effectively time exercise with fasting windows:

Morning Workouts During Fasting Window: Some women over 50 may prefer to exercise in the morning during their fasting window. This approach can help jumpstart metabolism, enhance fat burning, and promote mental clarity and focus throughout the day. Option for low to moderate-intensity activities such as walking, yoga, or light strength training to avoid overexertion on an empty stomach.

Low-Intensity Activities During Fasting:
Engage in low-intensity activities such as walking, gentle yoga, or tai chi during fasting periods. These activities can help burn calories, improve circulation, and promote mobility without causing excessive fatigue or hunger. They're also gentle on the digestive system and may complement the fasting state well.

Hydration and Electrolyte Balance:
Stay hydrated before, during, and after exercise sessions, especially when fasting. Drink plenty of water and consider adding electrolytes to maintain hydration and electrolyte balance. Electrolytes can help prevent dehydration, muscle cramps, and fatigue during workouts, particularly in a fasted state.

Post-Workout Nutrition Timing:
If you choose to exercise during fasting periods, plan your post-workout meal strategically to replenish glycogen stores and support muscle recovery. Aim to consume a balanced meal or snack

containing carbohydrates, protein, and healthy fats within your feeding window to optimize recovery and nutrient replenishment.

Afternoon or Evening Workouts
During Feeding Window:
Alternatively, some women may prefer to exercise later in the day during their feeding window. This allows for optimal fueling before and after workouts, which can enhance performance, endurance, and recovery. Choose a variety of activities based on personal preference and fitness goals, such as strength training, cardio, or group fitness classes.

Pre-Workout Fueling Options:
If exercising later in the day, consider consuming a small, balanced meal or snack containing carbohydrates and protein approximately 1-2 hours before your workout. This provides fuel for optimal performance and helps prevent blood sugar fluctuations during exercise. A turkey sandwich on whole grain bread, Greek yogurt with fruit, and bananas with nut butter are a few examples.

Listen to Your Body's Signals:
Pay attention to your body's signals and adjust your exercise timing and intensity based on how you feel. If you experience dizziness, weakness, or fatigue during fasted workouts, consider scaling back the intensity or switching to a different activity. Always prioritize safety and avoid pushing yourself beyond your limits.

Consistency and Adaptability:
Consistency is key when integrating exercise with intermittent fasting. Find a schedule and routine that works for you and stick to it consistently. However, be flexible and adaptable to changes in your energy levels, schedule, or preferences, and adjust your exercise timing as needed to ensure a sustainable and enjoyable fitness regimen.

By timing exercise strategically within fasting windows, women over 50 can optimize the benefits of both intermittent fasting and physical activity, leading to improved overall health, fitness, and well-being. Remember to prioritize hydration, proper nutrition, and listening to your body's cues to support optimal performance and recovery.

Maximizing Fitness and Weight Loss Results

Achieving optimal fitness and weight loss results with intermittent fasting requires a comprehensive approach tailored to the unique needs of women over 50. By combining smart dietary choices, effective exercise strategies, and lifestyle modifications, women can maximize their success in reaching their health and wellness goals. Here's a comprehensive guide on how to maximize fitness and weight loss results for women over 50 practicing intermittent fasting:

Set Realistic Goals:
Start by setting realistic and achievable goals that align with your age, lifestyle, and health status. Focus on goals related to improving overall health, increasing fitness levels, and achieving sustainable weight loss rather than solely focusing on the number on the scale.

Follow a Balanced Diet:

Adopt a balanced and nutritious diet that provides essential nutrients while supporting your weight loss and fitness goals. Emphasize whole foods such as fruits, vegetables, lean proteins, whole grains, and healthy fats, and limit processed foods, added sugars, and excessive calorie intake.

Practice Intermittent Fasting Consistently:

Follow an intermittent fasting schedule consistently to optimize its benefits for weight loss and metabolic health. Choose a fasting protocol that aligns with your lifestyle and preferences, such as the 16/8 method or the 14/10 method, and stick to it consistently over time.

Incorporate Exercise Regularly:

Engage in a variety of exercise modalities regularly to maximize fitness and weight loss results. Include cardiovascular exercise, strength training, flexibility work, and functional movements in your routine to target different aspects of fitness and support overall health and well-being.

Combine Cardio and Strength Training:
Incorporate both cardiovascular exercise and strength training into your workout routine to maximize calorie burn, improve muscle tone, and boost metabolism. Aim for a balanced approach that includes a mix of aerobic activities and resistance exercises to achieve optimal results.

Prioritize High-Intensity Interval Training (HIIT):
Consider adding high-intensity interval training (HIIT) to your exercise routine to maximize calorie burn, improve cardiovascular fitness, and stimulate fat loss. HIIT workouts involve short bursts of intense exercise followed by brief rest periods and can be an efficient and effective way to achieve fitness and weight loss goals.

Monitor Portion Sizes and Caloric Intake:
Pay attention to portion sizes and caloric intake, even when practicing intermittent fasting. While

fasting can help regulate appetite and reduce overall calorie intake, it's still essential to be mindful of portion sizes and avoid overeating during feeding windows to support weight loss goals.

Stay Hydrated and Manage Stress:
Prioritize hydration and stress management to support overall health and weight loss efforts. Drink plenty of water throughout the day, practice stress-reducing techniques such as meditation or deep breathing, and prioritize adequate sleep to optimize hormonal balance and metabolic function.

Listen to Your Body:
Pay attention to your body's signals and adjust your approach as needed based on how you feel. If you experience fatigue, hunger, or discomfort, make modifications to your fasting or exercise routine to ensure safety and well-being.

Seek Professional Guidance if Needed:
If you're struggling to achieve your fitness or weight loss goals, consider seeking guidance from a healthcare professional, registered dietitian, or certified fitness trainer who specializes in working with women over 50. They can provide

personalized recommendations, support, and accountability to help you reach your desired outcomes.

Synergies between Intermittent Fasting and Exercise

The combination of intermittent fasting and exercise can create powerful synergies for women over 50, leading to enhanced health, fitness, and overall well-being. When practiced together strategically, intermittent fasting and exercise can complement each other to optimize metabolic health, support weight management, and improve physical fitness. Here's a closer look at the synergies between intermittent fasting and exercise for women over 50:

Enhanced Fat Burning:
Intermittent fasting and exercise both promote fat burning, making them a potent combination for weight loss and body composition improvement. During fasting periods, the body taps into stored fat for energy, while exercise further stimulates fat

oxidation, especially when performed in a fasted state. This synergy can accelerate fat loss and help women over 50 achieve their weight loss goals more effectively.

Improved Insulin Sensitivity:
Both intermittent fasting and exercise have been shown to improve insulin sensitivity, which is crucial for managing blood sugar levels and reducing the risk of insulin resistance and type 2 diabetes. Intermittent fasting helps regulate insulin levels and enhance insulin sensitivity, while exercise enhances glucose uptake by muscles, leading to better blood sugar control. By combining the two, women over 50 can optimize their metabolic health and reduce the risk of chronic diseases associated with insulin resistance.

Muscle Preservation and Strength:
Intermittent fasting, when combined with resistance training, can help preserve lean muscle mass and promote strength gains, especially in women over 50 who may be at risk of age-related muscle loss (sarcopenia). Exercise stimulates muscle protein synthesis, while intermittent fasting helps preserve muscle by promoting the secretion of growth

hormone and reducing muscle breakdown. This synergy supports muscle maintenance, improves functional capacity, and enhances overall physical strength and vitality.

Optimized Hormonal Balance:
Both intermittent fasting and exercise influence hormonal balance in the body, leading to various health benefits for women over 50. Intermittent fasting can regulate hormones such as insulin, growth hormone, and cortisol, while exercise stimulates the release of endorphins and other feel-good hormones that promote mood, energy, and well-being. This synergy can help alleviate symptoms of hormonal imbalance, such as mood swings, fatigue, and metabolic dysfunction, and support overall hormonal health.

Increased Energy and Vitality:
Regular exercise, when combined with intermittent fasting, can increase energy levels and promote feelings of vitality and well-being in women over 50. Exercise boosts circulation, oxygenation, and nutrient delivery to tissues, while intermittent fasting enhances cellular repair and renewal processes. Together, they promote cellular energy

production, mitochondrial health, and overall vitality, leading to increased energy levels and improved resilience to stress and fatigue.

Enhanced Cognitive Function:
Both intermittent fasting and exercise have been shown to support cognitive function and brain health, which is particularly important for women over 50 seeking to maintain mental sharpness and cognitive vitality. Intermittent fasting promotes neuroplasticity, enhances brain-derived neurotrophic factor (BDNF) levels, and protects against age-related cognitive decline, while exercise increases cerebral blood flow, promotes neurogenesis, and enhances cognitive function. This synergy can help preserve cognitive function, memory, and mental clarity as women age.

Longevity and Aging Gracefully:
The synergistic effects of intermittent fasting and exercise extend beyond immediate health benefits and can contribute to longevity and aging gracefully for women over 50. Both practices have been associated with longevity-promoting pathways such

as autophagy, mitochondrial biogenesis, and cellular stress resistance.

By supporting cellular repair, reducing inflammation, and enhancing metabolic efficiency, intermittent fasting and exercise can promote healthy aging and improve overall quality of life in women over 50.

In summary, the combination of exercise and intermittent fasting has many health advantages for women over 50. These benefits include better insulin sensitivity, increased energy and vitality, better fat burning, preserved muscle mass and strength, improved hormonal balance, improved cognitive function, and support for long life and healthy aging. Women over fifty can maintain and improve their health, fitness, and general well-being for years to come by implementing both activities into their lifestyle in a sustainable and balanced manner.

Avoiding Overtraining and Injury

While exercise is important for overall health and well-being, women over 50 should approach it with caution to avoid overtraining and injury, especially when combined with intermittent fasting. Here are some important considerations to help women over 50 prevent overtraining and injury while practicing intermittent fasting:

Listen to Your Body:
Pay attention to your body's signals and avoid pushing yourself too hard, especially during fasted workouts. If you experience excessive fatigue, pain, dizziness, or other signs of overtraining or injury, take a break and allow your body time to rest and recover.

Gradually Increase Intensity:
Gradually increase the intensity and duration of your workouts to avoid overexertion and minimize

the risk of injury. Start with low to
moderate-intensity exercises and gradually progress
over time as your fitness level improves. Avoid
sudden increases in intensity or volume that can
place undue stress on your body.

Incorporate Rest Days:
Incorporate regular rest days into your workout
schedule to allow your body time to recover and
repair. Rest days are essential for preventing
overtraining, reducing the risk of injury, and
promoting overall recovery and adaptation to
exercise. Listen to your body's need for rest and
avoid exercising every day without adequate
recovery time.

Balance Different Types of Exercise:
Maintain a balanced approach to exercise by
incorporating a variety of activities that target
different muscle groups and energy systems.
Include a mix of cardiovascular exercise, strength
training, flexibility work, and low-impact activities
to avoid overuse injuries and promote overall
fitness and mobility.

Warm Up and Cool Down Properly:
Always warm up properly before starting your workout and cool down afterward to prevent injury and promote recovery. Warm-up exercises should include dynamic movements to increase blood flow and prepare your muscles and joints for activity. Cool-down activities such as stretching can help reduce muscle soreness and improve flexibility.

Pay Attention to Form and Technique:
Focus on proper form and technique during exercise to minimize the risk of injury and maximize the effectiveness of your workouts. If you're unsure about how to perform a specific exercise correctly, seek guidance from a qualified fitness professional or trainer.

Stay Hydrated and Well-Nourished:
Stay hydrated before, during, and after exercise, especially when fasting. Dehydration can increase the risk of injury and negatively impact

performance. Additionally, ensure you're consuming adequate nutrients and calories to support your energy needs and promote muscle repair and recovery.

Avoid Overexercise in a Fasted State:
While it's possible to exercise in a fasted state, be mindful of your energy levels and avoid overexertion. If you find that fasted workouts leave you feeling weak or fatigued, consider adjusting your exercise timing to coincide with your feeding window or consuming a small snack before exercising.

Modify Intensity and Frequency as Needed:
Be willing to modify your exercise intensity and frequency based on your body's response and feedback. If you're experiencing persistent fatigue, soreness, or signs of overtraining, scale back your workouts or take additional rest days to allow for recovery.

Consult with a Healthcare Professional:
If you're experiencing chronic pain, persistent injuries, or other health concerns related to exercise, consult with a healthcare professional or physical

therapist for evaluation and guidance. They can help diagnose any underlying issues, develop a tailored exercise plan, and provide recommendations for injury prevention and management.

CHAPTER EIGHT

Health Benefits Beyond Weight Loss

Intermittent fasting offers a multitude of health benefits beyond weight loss, especially for women over 50. While weight management is often a primary motivation for adopting intermittent fasting, the practice can positively impact various aspects of health and well-being. Here's a comprehensive overview of the health benefits beyond weight loss for women over 50 practicing intermittent fasting:

Improved Metabolic Health:
Intermittent fasting can improve metabolic health by enhancing insulin sensitivity, reducing inflammation, and promoting better blood sugar control. These effects are particularly beneficial for

women over 50 who may be at a higher risk of insulin resistance and metabolic syndrome.

Enhanced Cellular Repair and Autophagy:
Fasting triggers cellular repair processes such as autophagy, where cells remove damaged components and recycle them for energy. This rejuvenating effect can promote cellular health, longevity, and resilience, contributing to overall well-being and vitality.

Cardiovascular Health Benefits:
Intermittent fasting has been associated with improved cardiovascular health markers, including reduced blood pressure, improved cholesterol levels, and decreased markers of inflammation. These benefits can help lower the risk of heart disease, stroke, and other cardiovascular conditions, which become more prevalent with age.

Brain Health and Cognitive Function:

Intermittent fasting has neuroprotective effects and may help preserve cognitive function and brain health in women over 50. Studies suggest that fasting stimulates the production of brain-derived

neurotrophic factor (BDNF), a protein that supports the growth and maintenance of brain cells, potentially reducing the risk of age-related cognitive decline and neurodegenerative diseases such as Alzheimer's.

Increased Human Growth Hormone (HGH) Production:
Intermittent fasting can stimulate the production of human growth hormone (HGH), which plays a role in metabolism, muscle growth, and cellular repair. Higher levels of HGH may promote muscle preservation, fat loss, and overall vitality in women over 50.

Reduction in Chronic Inflammation:
Chronic inflammation is associated with various age-related diseases, including arthritis, heart

disease, and cognitive decline. Intermittent fasting has been shown to reduce markers of inflammation in the body, which can help mitigate the risk of chronic diseases and support overall health and longevity.

Enhanced Immune Function:
Intermittent fasting may support immune function by promoting the production of white blood cells, reducing inflammation, and enhancing cellular repair mechanisms. A healthy immune system is essential for defending against infections and illnesses, particularly as women age and immune function naturally declines.

Potential Cancer-Protective Effects:
Some research suggests that intermittent fasting may have cancer-protective effects by inhibiting tumor growth, reducing inflammation, and promoting cellular repair and apoptosis (programmed cell death). While more studies are needed to fully understand the relationship between fasting and cancer risk, the potential benefits are

promising for women over 50 seeking to reduce their risk of cancer.

Longevity and Aging Gracefully:
By promoting metabolic health, cellular repair, and resilience to stress, intermittent fasting has the potential to support longevity and healthy aging in women over 50. While aging is inevitable, adopting lifestyle practices such as intermittent fasting can help optimize healthspan and improve quality of life as women age.

Improved Gut Health and Digestive Function:
Intermittent fasting may support gut health by promoting gut motility, microbial diversity, and digestive efficiency. Periods of fasting allow the digestive system to rest and repair, potentially improving symptoms of digestive disorders such as bloating, gas, and indigestion.

In summary, intermittent fasting offers numerous health benefits beyond weight loss for women over

50, including improved metabolic health, enhanced cellular repair, cardiovascular benefits, brain health and cognitive function, increased human growth hormone production, reduction in chronic inflammation, enhanced immune function, potential cancer-protective effects, longevity, and improved gut health.

Cognitive Health

As women age, maintaining cognitive health becomes increasingly important for overall well-being and quality of life. Intermittent fasting has emerged as a potential strategy to support cognitive function and brain health, offering numerous benefits for women over 50. Here's a comprehensive overview of how intermittent fasting can positively impact cognitive health in this demographic:

Preservation of Brain Function:
Intermittent fasting has been shown to support the preservation of brain function by promoting neuroplasticity, the brain's ability to reorganize and form new neural connections. This can help

mitigate age-related cognitive decline and maintain
cognitive function in women over 50.

Enhanced Neuroprotection:
Fasting triggers biochemical pathways that promote
neuroprotection, protecting brain cells from
oxidative stress, inflammation, and damage. These
neuroprotective effects can help reduce the risk of
neurodegenerative diseases such as Alzheimer's and
Parkinson's, which become more prevalent with
age.

**Stimulation of Brain-Derived
Neurotrophic Factor (BDNF):**
Intermittent fasting stimulates the production of
brain-derived neurotrophic factor (BDNF), a protein
that supports the growth, survival, and maintenance
of brain cells. Higher levels of BDNF are associated
with improved cognitive function, memory, and
learning, making intermittent fasting potentially
beneficial for cognitive health in women over 50.

Improved Memory and Learning:
Animal studies have shown that intermittent fasting can enhance memory and learning by promoting the growth of new neurons and synapses in the hippocampus, the brain region responsible for memory formation and spatial navigation. These findings suggest that intermittent fasting may support cognitive function and memory retention in women over 50.

Reduction of Neuroinflammation:
Chronic inflammation in the brain is implicated in the development of neurodegenerative diseases and cognitive decline. Intermittent fasting has anti-inflammatory effects and can help reduce neuroinflammation, potentially protecting against cognitive impairment and preserving brain health in women over 50.

Promotion of Autophagy and Cellular Repair:
Fasting induces autophagy, a cellular process that removes damaged components and recycles them for energy. This cellular cleanup process can help clear toxic protein aggregates and dysfunctional mitochondria from brain cells, promoting neuronal health and longevity.

Enhanced Cognitive Flexibility:
Intermittent fasting may enhance cognitive flexibility, the ability to adapt and switch between different tasks or mental processes. This cognitive benefit can support problem-solving, decision-making, and overall mental agility in women over 50, contributing to better cognitive function and resilience.

Mitigation of Age-Related Cognitive Decline:
By promoting neuroprotection, neuroplasticity, and cellular repair, intermittent fasting has the potential to mitigate age-related cognitive decline and maintain cognitive function in women over 50. While aging is inevitable, adopting lifestyle practices such as intermittent fasting can help optimize cognitive health and promote cognitive vitality as women age.

Potential Protection Against

Neurodegenerative Diseases:
Some research suggests that intermittent fasting
may offer protection against neurodegenerative
diseases such as Alzheimer's and Parkinson's by
reducing risk factors such as oxidative stress,
inflammation, and protein aggregation. While more
studies are needed to fully understand the
relationship between fasting and neurodegenerative
diseases, the potential benefits are promising for
women over 50 seeking to preserve cognitive
health.

Improved Mood and Mental Well-Being:
Intermittent fasting has been associated with
improvements in mood, stress resilience, and mental
well-being, which are important factors for overall
cognitive health and quality of life in women over
50. By promoting neurochemical balance and stress

resilience, intermittent fasting may contribute to better mood regulation and mental resilience as women age.

Heart Health

Maintaining heart health becomes increasingly crucial as women age, especially for those over 50 who may be at a higher risk of cardiovascular disease. Intermittent fasting has gained attention for its potential to support heart health by improving various cardiovascular risk factors. Here's a comprehensive overview of how intermittent fasting can positively impact heart health in women over 50:

Improved Blood Pressure Regulation:
Intermittent fasting has been shown to help regulate blood pressure levels, reducing the risk of hypertension, a major risk factor for heart disease. By promoting better blood pressure control,

intermittent fasting may contribute to overall heart health in women over 50.

Reduction in LDL Cholesterol Levels:
Intermittent fasting may lead to a decrease in LDL cholesterol levels, often referred to as "bad" cholesterol. High levels of LDL cholesterol are associated with an increased risk of atherosclerosis and coronary artery disease.

By lowering LDL cholesterol levels, intermittent fasting may help reduce the risk of cardiovascular events in women over 50.

Increase in HDL Cholesterol Levels:
Intermittent fasting has been shown to increase HDL cholesterol levels, often referred to as "good" cholesterol. HDL cholesterol helps remove LDL cholesterol from the bloodstream, reducing the risk of plaque buildup in the arteries. Higher levels of HDL cholesterol are associated with improved heart health and reduced risk of cardiovascular disease.

Enhanced Insulin Sensitivity:
Intermittent fasting improves insulin sensitivity, which is crucial for maintaining stable blood sugar levels and reducing the risk of insulin resistance and

type 2 diabetes. By enhancing insulin sensitivity, intermittent fasting may help prevent diabetes-related complications and reduce the risk of heart disease in women over 50.

Reduction in Inflammation:
Chronic inflammation is a key contributor to the development of cardiovascular disease. Intermittent fasting has anti-inflammatory effects, reducing levels of inflammatory markers such as C-reactive protein (CRP) and interleukin-6 (IL-6). By lowering inflammation, intermittent fasting may help protect against heart disease and promote cardiovascular health in women over 50.
Promotion of Weight Loss and

Weight Management:
Intermittent fasting can aid in weight loss and weight management, which are important factors for heart health. Excess weight, particularly around the abdomen, is associated with an increased risk of heart disease, hypertension, and other

cardiovascular conditions. By promoting weight loss and reducing body fat, intermittent fasting may help improve heart health in women over 50.

Enhanced Autophagy and Cellular Repair:
Fasting stimulates autophagy, a cellular process that removes damaged components and promotes cellular repair and renewal. This cellular cleanup process may help protect against age-related changes in the heart and blood vessels, supporting cardiovascular health in women over 50.

Optimized Lipid Profile:
Intermittent fasting has been shown to optimize lipid profiles by reducing triglyceride levels and improving the ratio of total cholesterol to HDL cholesterol. These improvements in lipid profile are associated with a lower risk of cardiovascular disease and may contribute to better heart health in women over 50.

Reduction in Oxidative Stress:

Intermittent fasting can reduce oxidative stress, which occurs when there is an imbalance between free radicals and antioxidants in the body. Oxidative stress is implicated in the development of cardiovascular disease and endothelial dysfunction. By reducing oxidative stress, intermittent fasting may help protect against heart disease and promote cardiovascular health in women over 50.

Improved Endothelial Function:
Endothelial dysfunction, characterized by impaired blood vessel function, is a hallmark of cardiovascular disease. Intermittent fasting has been shown to improve endothelial function, enhancing blood flow and vascular health. By promoting endothelial health, intermittent fasting may help reduce the risk of heart disease and support cardiovascular function in women over 50.

In summary, intermittent fasting offers numerous benefits for heart health in women over 50, including improved blood pressure regulation, reduction in LDL cholesterol levels, increase in HDL cholesterol levels, enhanced insulin sensitivity, reduction in inflammation, promotion of weight loss and weight management, enhanced autophagy and cellular repair, optimized lipid profile, reduction in oxidative stress, and improved endothelial function. By incorporating intermittent fasting into their lifestyle in a balanced and sustainable manner, women over 50 can optimize their heart health and reduce their risk of cardiovascular disease for years to come.

Managing Chronic Conditions

For women over 50 managing chronic conditions, incorporating intermittent fasting into their lifestyle can be a beneficial strategy to improve overall health and well-being. While intermittent fasting is not a cure-all, it may help manage certain chronic conditions and alleviate symptoms associated with aging. Here's a comprehensive guide on managing chronic conditions for women over 50 practicing intermittent fasting:

Consult with Healthcare Professionals:
Before starting intermittent fasting or making any significant changes to your diet or lifestyle, consult with healthcare professionals, including your primary care physician and any specialists managing your chronic conditions. They can

provide personalized recommendations and guidance based on your medical history, current health status, and individual needs.

Understand Potential Benefits and Risks:
Educate yourself about the potential benefits and risks of intermittent fasting, particularly in relation to your specific chronic conditions. While intermittent fasting may offer benefits such as improved metabolic health and weight management, it's essential to consider how fasting may affect your condition and any medications you're taking.

Monitor Blood Sugar Levels:
If you have diabetes or prediabetes, monitor your blood sugar levels closely while practicing intermittent fasting. Intermittent fasting can affect blood sugar levels, so it's important to work with your healthcare team to adjust your medication regimen and monitor for any fluctuations in blood sugar control.

Adjust Medications and Treatment Plans:

Work with your healthcare team to adjust your medications and treatment plans as needed while practicing intermittent fasting. Depending on your condition and individual response to fasting, your healthcare provider may need to modify your medication dosages or timing to ensure optimal management of your chronic conditions.

Stay Hydrated and Well-Nourished:
Maintain adequate hydration and nutrition during fasting periods to support overall health and well-being, especially if you have conditions such as hypertension or kidney disease. Drink plenty of water and consume nutrient-dense foods during feeding windows to ensure you're meeting your body's hydration and nutritional needs.

Monitor Symptoms and Listen to Your Body:
Pay attention to any changes in symptoms or how you feel while practicing intermittent fasting. If you experience any adverse effects such as dizziness, weakness, or exacerbation of chronic condition symptoms, stop fasting and consult with your healthcare provider.

Emphasize Nutrient-Dense Foods:

Focus on consuming nutrient-dense foods during feeding windows to provide essential vitamins, minerals, and antioxidants that support overall health and immune function. Include a variety of fruits, vegetables, lean proteins, whole grains, and healthy fats in your meals to optimize nutrition and manage chronic conditions effectively.

Manage Medication Timing:
If you take medications that require food or specific timing, work with your healthcare provider to adjust your medication schedule to align with your intermittent fasting protocol. This may involve taking medications with meals during feeding windows or adjusting dosages to accommodate fasting periods.

Consider Modified Fasting Approaches:
Depending on your individual health needs and preferences, consider modified fasting approaches that allow for more flexibility and customization. For example, time-restricted eating with a slightly longer feeding window or alternate-day fasting with fewer fasting days per week may be more suitable for managing chronic conditions while still reaping the benefits of intermittent fasting.

Monitor Progress and Seek Support:
Regularly monitor your progress, including changes
in symptoms, weight, blood sugar levels, and
overall well-being, while practicing intermittent
fasting. If you have any concerns or questions, don't
hesitate to seek support from your healthcare team,
dietitian, or other qualified professionals who can
provide guidance and assistance.

In summary, managing chronic conditions for
women over 50 practicing intermittent fasting
requires careful planning, monitoring, and
collaboration with healthcare professionals. By
understanding the potential benefits and risks,
adjusting medications and treatment plans as
needed, staying hydrated and well-nourished,
monitoring symptoms, emphasizing nutrient-dense
foods, managing medication timing, considering
modified fasting approaches, and seeking support

when necessary, women over 50 can effectively manage their chronic conditions while incorporating intermittent fasting into their lifestyle. With proper guidance and monitoring, intermittent fasting can be a valuable tool for improving overall health and well-being in women over 50 with chronic conditions.

Sample Meal Plans and Recipes

Creating balanced and nutritious meal plans is essential for women over 50 practicing intermittent fasting to ensure they meet their nutritional needs while supporting their health goals. Here are sample meal plans and recipes tailored for women over 50 incorporating intermittent fasting:

Sample Meal Plan: 16/8 Method

Feeding Window: 12:00 PM - 8:00 PM

Breakfast (12:00 PM):

Spinach and Feta Omelette:

Ingredients: Spinach, eggs, feta cheese, cherry tomatoes, olive oil.

Instructions: Saute spinach and cherry tomatoes in olive oil, then add beaten eggs and crumbled feta cheese. Cook until eggs are set, then fold over into an omelet.

Lunch (3:00 PM):

Grilled Chicken Salad:

Ingredients: Grilled chicken breast, mixed greens, cherry tomatoes, cucumber, avocado, balsamic vinaigrette.
Instructions: Combine grilled chicken breast with mixed greens, sliced cucumber, cherry tomatoes, and avocado. Drizzle with balsamic vinaigrette.

Snack (5:00 PM):

Greek Yogurt Parfait:

Ingredients: Greek yogurt, mixed berries, almonds, honey.

Instructions: Layer Greek yogurt with mixed berries and almonds in a glass, drizzle with honey.

Dinner (7:00 PM):

Baked Salmon with Roasted Vegetables:

Ingredients: Salmon filet, asparagus, bell peppers, zucchini, olive oil, lemon, garlic, herbs.
Instructions: Season salmon with olive oil, lemon juice, minced garlic, and herbs. Place on a baking sheet with asparagus, bell peppers, and zucchini. Bake until salmon is cooked through and vegetables are tender.

Sample Recipe: Mediterranean Quinoa Salad

Ingredients:
1 cup quinoa, rinsed
2 cups water or vegetable broth

1 cucumber, diced
1 pint cherry tomatoes, halved
1/2 red onion, finely chopped
1/4 cup Kalamata olives, pitted and sliced
1/4 cup crumbled feta cheese
2 tablespoons extra virgin olive oil

2 tablespoons lemon juice
1 teaspoon dried oregano
Salt and pepper to taste
Fresh parsley for garnish

Instructions:

- In a medium pot, combine quinoa with water or vegetable broth. After bringing to a boil, lower the heat to a simmer, cover, and cook the quinoa for 15 to 20 minutes, or until the liquid is absorbed. Remove from heat and let cool.
- In a large mixing bowl, combine cooked quinoa with diced cucumber, cherry tomatoes, red onion, Kalamata olives, and crumbled feta cheese.

- To make the dressing, combine the olive oil, lemon juice, dried oregano, salt, and pepper in a small bowl.
- Pour the dressing over the quinoa salad and toss to coat evenly.
- Garnish with fresh parsley before serving. Enjoy as a light and refreshing meal or side dish.

Tips for Meal Planning:
- Incorporate a range of nutrient-dense foods into your meals, including whole grains, fruits, vegetables, lean meats, and healthy fats.
- Prioritize hydration by drinking plenty of water throughout the day, especially during fasting periods.
- Experiment with different flavors, cuisines, and cooking methods to keep meals interesting and enjoyable.
- Listen to your body's hunger and fullness cues, and adjust portion sizes accordingly to meet your energy needs.

By following balanced meal plans and incorporating nutritious recipes like the ones provided above, women over 50 can support their health and well-being while practicing intermittent fasting. Remember to consult with healthcare professionals or registered dietitians for personalized guidance and recommendations based on individual health needs and goals.

Breakfast, Lunch, Dinner, and Snack Ideas

Breakfast Ideas:

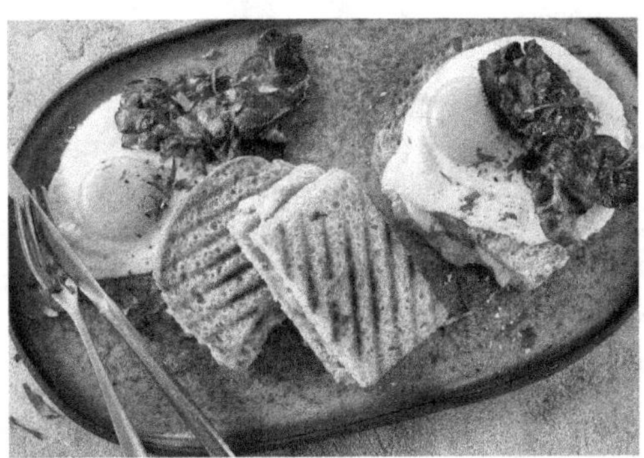

- **Greek Yogurt Parfait**: Layer Greek yogurt with mixed berries, granola, and a drizzle of honey for a satisfying and nutritious breakfast.
- **Veggie Omelet:** Cook a fluffy omelet filled with spinach, bell peppers, onions, and feta cheese for a protein-packed start to your day.

- **Overnight Oats**: Prepare overnight oats with rolled oats, almond milk, chia seeds, and sliced bananas. Customize with your favorite toppings such as nuts, seeds, or nut butter.
- **Avocado Toast**: Top whole-grain toast with mashed avocado, sliced tomatoes, and a sprinkle of feta cheese or Everything bagel seasoning for a quick and delicious breakfast option.
- **Smoothie Bowl**: Blend frozen berries, spinach, banana, Greek yogurt, and almond milk until smooth, then top with granola,

sliced fruit, and shredded coconut for a refreshing breakfast bowl.

Lunch Ideas:

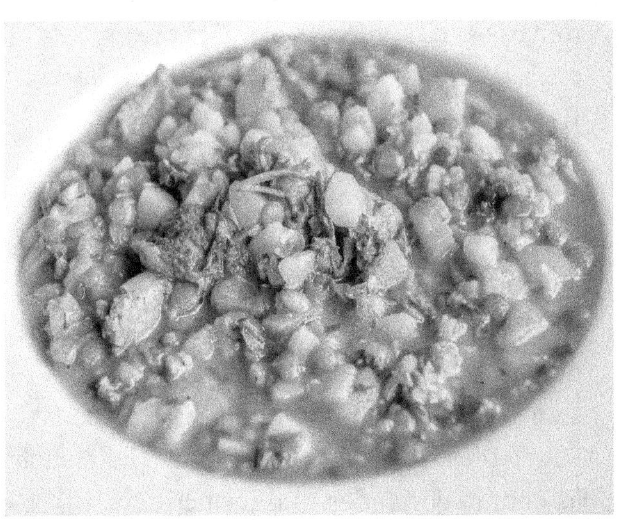

- **Quinoa Salad:** Combine cooked quinoa with diced cucumber, cherry tomatoes, bell peppers, black beans, corn, and a squeeze of lime juice for a vibrant and satisfying salad.
- **Turkey and Avocado Wrap**: Fill a whole-grain wrap with sliced turkey breast, avocado, lettuce, tomato, and mustard for a wholesome and portable lunch option.

- **Mediterranean Chickpea Salad:** Toss chickpeas with diced cucumber, cherry tomatoes, red onion, Kalamata olives, feta cheese, and a lemon-herb vinaigrette for a flavorful and filling salad.

- **Veggie Stir-Fry**: Stir-fry mixed vegetables such as broccoli, bell peppers, snap peas, and carrots with tofu or shrimp and a savory sauce. Serve over brown rice or quinoa for a nutritious lunch.
- **Lentil Soup:** Simmer lentils with diced vegetables, vegetable broth, and spices such as cumin, coriander, and turmeric for a

hearty and comforting soup that's packed with fiber and protein.

Dinner Ideas:

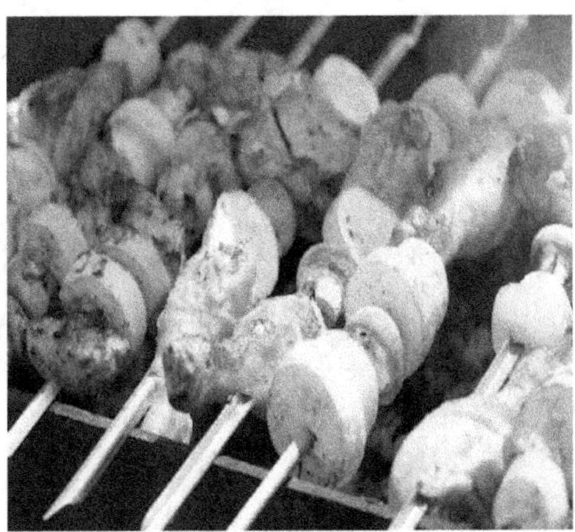

- **Baked Salmon with Roasted Vegetables:** Season salmon filets with olive oil, lemon juice, and herbs, then bake until flaky. Serve with roasted vegetables such as asparagus, carrots, and Brussels sprouts for a nutritious and flavorful dinner.

- **Chicken and Vegetable Skewers:** Thread chicken breast cubes, cherry tomatoes, bell peppers, onions, and mushrooms onto skewers, then grill or bake until cooked through. Serve with a side of quinoa or couscous for a balanced meal.

- **Veggie Stir-Fried Noodles:** Stir-fry soba noodles with tofu or tempeh, broccoli, bell peppers, snap peas, and carrots in a flavorful sauce made from soy sauce, garlic, ginger, and sesame oil for a delicious and satisfying dinner.

- **Stuffed Bell Peppers:** Fill halved bell peppers with a mixture of cooked quinoa, black beans, corn, diced tomatoes, and spices, then bake until tender. Top with avocado slices and salsa for a tasty and nutritious meal.

- **Grilled Veggie and Halloumi Salad**: Grill slices of halloumi cheese along with zucchini, eggplant, and red onion until charred and tender. Serve over mixed greens with a balsamic vinaigrette for a light and summery dinner option.

Snack Ideas:

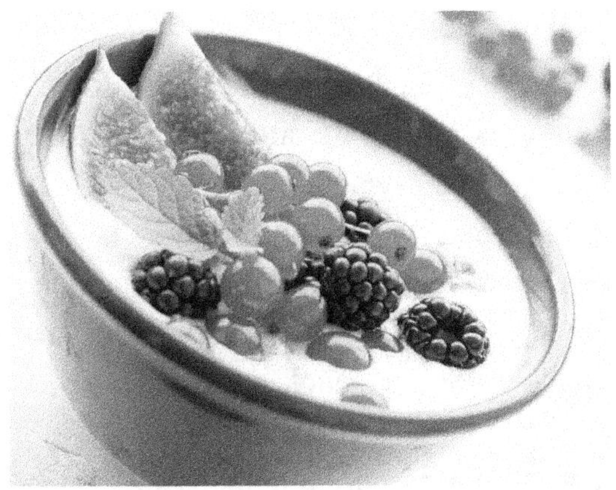

Greek Yogurt with Berries

- **Hummus and Veggie Sticks**: Dip carrot, cucumber, and bell pepper sticks into hummus for a satisfying and nutritious snack.
- **Greek Yogurt with Berries**: Top a bowl of Greek yogurt with fresh berries and a sprinkle of granola or nuts for a protein-rich snack.

- **Apple Slices with Almond Butter**: Spread almond butter onto apple slices for a crunchy and satisfying snack that combines protein, healthy fats, and fiber.
- **Trail Mix**: Mix together nuts, seeds, dried fruit, and dark chocolate chips for a portable and energy-boosting snack.
- **Rice Cake with Avocado**: Spread mashed avocado onto a rice cake and top with sliced cucumber, radish, and a sprinkle of sea salt for a quick and tasty snack option.

These breakfast, lunch, dinner, and snack ideas provide a variety of delicious and nutritious options for women over 50 practicing intermittent fasting. Remember to listen to your body's hunger and fullness cues, and choose foods that nourish your body and support your health goals.

CONCLUSION

Intermittent fasting has emerged as a powerful lifestyle approach for women over 50 seeking to optimize their health, vitality, and overall well-being. Through the strategic alternation of fasting periods and feeding windows, intermittent fasting offers a holistic approach to health that aligns with the unique needs and goals of women in this demographic. As we conclude our exploration of intermittent fasting for women over 50, it's important to reflect on the myriad benefits, considerations, and implications of this dietary practice.

First and foremost, intermittent fasting holds immense promise as a tool for promoting metabolic health and weight management in women over 50. By regulating blood sugar levels, enhancing insulin sensitivity, and promoting fat metabolism, intermittent fasting can support healthy weight loss and weight maintenance goals, helping women achieve greater metabolic efficiency and balance as they age.

Moreover, intermittent fasting has been shown to offer cardiovascular benefits, including improvements in blood pressure regulation, cholesterol levels, and heart health markers. For women over 50 at an increased risk of cardiovascular disease, these benefits are particularly significant, offering a natural and accessible means of reducing risk factors and promoting heart health.

Beyond its metabolic and cardiovascular benefits, intermittent fasting holds promise for supporting cognitive function and brain health in women over 50. Through mechanisms such as the stimulation of

brain-derived neurotrophic factor (BDNF),
reduction of neuroinflammation, and enhancement
of cellular repair processes, intermittent fasting may
help mitigate age-related cognitive decline, preserve
brain function, and promote cognitive vitality as
women age. Additionally, intermittent fasting has
been associated with improvements in mood, stress
resilience, and emotional well-being, providing
women over 50 with holistic support for mental
health and overall quality of life.

However, it's important to recognize that
intermittent fasting is not a one-size-fits-all
approach, and individual experiences may vary.
Women over 50 should approach intermittent
fasting with mindfulness, self-awareness, and a
willingness to adapt their approach based on their
unique needs, preferences, and health
considerations. Consulting with healthcare
professionals, including physicians, dietitians, and
other qualified practitioners, can provide invaluable
guidance and support in navigating the intermittent
fasting journey and optimizing health outcomes.

In conclusion, intermittent fasting holds immense
promise as a holistic approach to health and

wellness for women over 50. By embracing the principles of intermittent fasting, women in this demographic can harness the transformative power of fasting to support metabolic health, cardiovascular function, cognitive vitality, and overall well-being. Through mindfulness, self-reflection, and a commitment to personalized health goals, women over 50 can start on a journey of empowerment, resilience, and vitality as they embrace intermittent fasting as a cornerstone of their health and wellness journey.